The Handicapped Child

The Handicapped Child

ASSESSMENT AND
MANAGEMENT

GRACE E. WOODS

MB, BS, MD, MRCPsych, DPH, DCH
Consultant Paediatrician
(Handicapped Children),
Seacroft Hospital and
St James's Hospital, Leeds

BLACKWELL SCIENTIFIC PUBLICATIONS

OXFORD LONDON EDINBURGH MELBOURNE

© 1975 Blackwell Scientific Publications
Osney Mead, Oxford
85 Marylebone High Street, London W1
9 Forrest Road, Edinburgh
PO Box 9, North Balwyn, Victoria, Australia

ISBN 0 632 00481 9

First published 1975

Distributed in the United States of America
by J.B.Lippincott Company, Philadelphia
and in Canada by
J.B.Lippincott Company of
Canada Ltd, Toronto

Set by Santype Ltd, Salisbury and
Printed in Great Britain by
Whitstable Litho Ltd
Whitstable, Kent

Contents

vi   *Contents*

Preface

The purpose of this book is to pass on knowledge about handicapped children to doctors who, at different times in the child's life, are asked to supervise medical care and treatment. The family doctor or doctor in an infant welfare clinic may be the first medical person consulted by the parent of a handicapped child. Family doctors and school medical officers have the responsibility of ensuring an adequate service for the handicapped child during school life. The medical officer who advises on the placement of the handicapped adolescent in employment, and the clinician who supervises the adult handicapped since childhood, should have an appreciation of the clinical conditions responsible for the handicap, and the effect it has had on the early life of the child.

But the overall responsibility for clinical assessment and care is in the hands of the paediatrician, and it is hoped this book will be used as a textbook by the paediatric house officer and registrar, who later as a paediatrician may be the key medical person looking after the handicapped child. Details of biochemical, electromyographic and other investigations are not included as these may be found in the more general paediatric textbooks available.

Acknowledgments

Throughout the preparation of this book, I have drawn on the experience of colleagues from a number of special centres. I am particularly indebted to the staff at the Centre for Spastic Children, Cheyne Walk, Chelsea, London, for their advice and information on treatment and appliances and for the use of photographs. I am grateful to the Headmaster and staff of The Marjory Kinnon School, Hounslow, Middlesex, for allowing me to use material from a survey of clinical conditions in children who are educationally subnormal. I was fortunate to receive the help of Miss Catherine Renfrew of the Speech Therapy Department, Churchill Hospital, Oxford, in the chapter on speech disorders.

I should like to thank the several colleagues who have read parts of the text and given me the benefit of their advice. I should also like to thank the men and women of Bristol whom I knew a good many years ago and who were willing to let me use photographs of them as children.

Chapter 1
Introduction

Definition

A physically handicapped child may be defined as a child who is unable to lead the normal life of a child for a prolonged period due to a crippling organic illness.

Sheridan's (1962) definition, which was adopted by the Sheldon Committee (1967) enquiring into the need for assessment centres for the handicapped child, describes a handicapped child as 'a child suffering from any continuing disability of body, intellect or personality likely to interfere with his normal growth, development and capacity to learn.' This book considers children with a handicap due to a condition which is presumed to have an organic pathology.

Incidence

It is difficult to give exact figures on the incidence of handicapping conditions in children. The figure of 4 per 1000 live births is generally accepted as the incidence of mental subnormality (IQ below 50). Two per 1000 is an estimate of the incidence of cerebral palsy, of which 0·5 to 1 per 1000 may be also mentally subnormal. The incidence of spina bifida is variously estimated as about 0·5 to 3 per 1000. Blindness and a severe hearing loss are in the region of 1·7 per 10,000 school children and 4·2 per 10,000 respectively. The incidence of educational subnormality in children (IQ 50–70) has been conservatively estimated as between 1% and 3% of all children. Figures for other handicaps such as autism, minimal cerebral dysfunction, partial sight, depend very much on definition of the condition, and the enthusiasm with which cases are investigated in any community. The overall figure for organically handicapped children in the total school population is likely to be above 3%.

Change in Type of Handicap

In the past, handicapped children who came to the notice of health and education authorities were children whose handicap was caused by a single insult to a normal child—deafness due to otitis media, blindness due to neonatal infection, muscle weakness due to anterior poliomyelitis, cardiac insufficiency due to rheumatic fever, and defects in locomotion due to tuberculosis of bone or osteomyelitis. These conditions comprise only a very small percentage of the causes of childhood handicap today in countries with preventive health services.

Conditions that may have caused infantile deaths in the past, or were considered too severe for educational help, are now coming to the fore. The diseases which cause major handicaps today may be genetic in origin; or caused by biochemical or infective damage to the developing fetus; or due to perinatal or neonatal illness; or due to trauma or infection in childhood.

Often damage involves the central nervous system. Sight, hearing, movement, speech, sensory and cognitive functions and intelligence may be affected to varying degrees. This means that the majority of handicapped children today are multiple handicapped. The individual handicaps are also complex in nature. Visual defect may be due to disorder of the field of vision or of eye movements, to refractive errors, or damage to the nerve pathways leading to the occipital cortex, which affects the child's ability to interpret the images projected on to the retina. Speech defect may be due to varying forms of deafness, a receptive, executive or central communication disorder, or a motor disorder of the muscles of speech.

Variety of Handicaps

In attempting to discuss the various types of handicaps in separate chapters, one is well aware that as far as the multiple handicapped child is concerned, this division is largely artificial. Nevertheless it is important to define the major handicap—blindness or severe hearing loss—as this determines the type of education which the child will receive. It is hoped that schools catering for a particular handicap will have facilities to deal with children with additional handicaps.

Paediatrician and Team Approach

The clinical care of the handicapped child must be the overall responsibility of the paediatrician both in the early assessment, support and guidance to parents, and in the supervision of treatment. This involves working closely with therapists and understanding their methods.

Training and education are the province of teachers and psychologists, and the problems of the family and of daily living are the concern of the social services. Very little effective help can be given unless the paediatrician leads the team in every matter concerning the clinical welfare of the child and takes an active interest in the work of these other departments. The medical duties of the paediatrician dovetail with those of the educationist and social worker.

Throughout this book, school placement is mentioned repeatedly. Doctors caring for handicapped children must work closely with teachers and be active members of the staff of schools for the handicapped. It has been said that when a visitor enters one of these schools and sees two doors, one labelled *Headmaster* and the other *Medical Officer*, he knows it is a good school. A school for handicapped children cannot function satisfactorily unless a medical expert for that particular handicap is generally available, a fact proved conclusively in the schools for the cerebral palsied. Many head teachers actively interested in the children's welfare bemoan the lack of this expert help. The paediatrician must go into the school.

Educationists and psychologists working in university departments and special schools and hospitals have contributed a vast amount of new knowledge in the last few years about learning difficulties and visual and communication problems, which can be used in the training of the child whether he is mentally severely subnormal, deaf, blind, or cerebral palsied. Much of this specialised work is outside the field of the paediatrician, but it is important he knows it is going on, understands the basic principles, and uses his influence in the team to see that all new knowledge is applied to the training of the handicapped child.

Chapter 2
Early Assessment of the Handicapped Child

Referral

Parents with a handicapped child usually start to worry about the child's slowness in development during the first year of life. This is true of children with defective sight or hearing, cerebral palsy and mental retardation. Parents may notice that a child is not as responsive as he should be when there is a later handicap such as autism, marked language delay, or an intelligence quotient in the range 50–70. Many parents will approach the family doctor or health visitor at this early age and the parents' concern should be taken seriously. Ideally all handicapped children should be referred to a paediatrician at an early age.

'At Risk' Register

Many administrative areas in the United Kingdom and in other parts of the world run an 'at risk' register, first suggested by Sheridan (1962), on which the names of babies who, for one reason or another, are at a greater risk than normal of being handicapped, are placed at birth for special follow-up. The list includes the following categories.

Genetic

1 Family history (parents, brothers or sisters) of congenital deafness, blindness, mental disorder, etc.

Prenatal

2 Virus infections—rubella or hepatitis in first 3 months of pregnancy
3 Diabetes

4

4 Illnesses necessitating the use of the following drugs in pregnancy—thyroid and antithyroid drugs, progesterone and androgens, cortisone, streptomycin
5 Abdominal or pelvic X-ray
6 Rhesus sensitisation
7 Any uterine bleeding
8 Toxaemia occurring in the last 3 months of pregnancy
9 Mother over 40 years of age

Perinatal

10 Abnormal or assisted delivery—breech, forceps, Caesarian
11 Multiple pregnancy
12 Birth weight under $5\frac{1}{2}$ lb
13 Birth anoxia (blue or white colour, with limp or absent muscle tone). Low Apgar score
14 Fetal distress

Postnatal

15 Jaundice
16 Convulsions
17 Respiratory distress, cyanotic attacks
18 Any congenital abnormalities that may be a handicap to the individual
19 Maternal puerperal psychosis, or any psychiatric condition warranting consultant opinion
20 Failure to thrive

In practice it is found that a high proportion of children eventually found to be handicapped are on these lists. This is particularly true of children who are handicapped following birth abnormality, prematurity, perinatal or neonatal illness.

Routine Follow-up

Children on the 'at risk' register should be seen at the ages of 1 month, 3 months, 7 months, 1 year and each 6 months after that until they enter primary school.

Table 2.1 gives suggested tests for each age, and in practice has

Table 2.1

Age	Test
ONE MONTH	Tone of muscle Rooting reflex Moro reflex Stepping reflex Grasp reflex Light shone into eyes Small bell rung or voice cooing at ear Watches mother's face when she is talking to him
THREE MONTHS	Holds back straight and head erect—5 seconds Visually follows moving object through 180° Stares at mother when feeding Smiles and coos in response to friendly adult Hand-eye regard developing, waves hands apart and together Quick response to bell rung 3–5 seconds 6–12 inches from ear
SEVEN MONTHS	Lifts head from pillow Sits alone 10–15 minutes Rolls over—from front to back Bounces when feet on firm surface Attempts to crawl Palmar grasp Passes object from hand to hand Babbling (single syllables) Responds to Stycar hearing tests Shakes rattle deliberately
TWELVE MONTHS	Crawls rapidly and shuffles Pulls himself up to stand holding on Walks with support Drops toys deliberately and watches them Picks up objects with precise pincer grasp Uses both hands but often prefers one Drinks from cup with help Says a few syllables and words—ma-ma, da-da, wo-wo (vocalising) Waves bye-bye Knows his name and comprehends simple requests Rings bell and pokes at clapper

Table 2.1—*Continued*

EIGHTEEN MONTHS	Walks and runs
	Walks upstairs with one hand held
	Picks up small objects from floor without falling
	Builds tower of three cubes
	Holds cup with two hands and drinks with a little spilling
	Shows own hair, nose, eyes, pointing to parts of body
TWO YEARS	Runs safely
	Walks up and down stairs independently
	Throws small ball
	Builds tower of six cubes
	Spontaneous circular scribble
	Spoon-feed without spilling
	Puts two words together and makes simple phrases
	Asks for potty
	Bowel control often attained
	Plays near but not with other children
TWO AND HALF YEARS	Stands on tip-toe
	Builds tower of seven to eight blocks
	Copies line and circle
	Knows name and sex
	Uses pronouns in place of own name
THREE YEARS	Stands momentarily on one leg
	Cuts with scissors
	Builds bridge of three cubes
	Sheridan five-letter charts
	Talks clearly in sentences
	Washes hands but needs help with drying
	Dry at night
	Plays with and takes turn with other children
FOUR YEARS	Can hop on one foot
	Single-letter vision test at 10 feet
	(Sheridan charts seven letters)
	Copies cross
	Gives home address
	General behaviour self-willed, imaginative play

been found helpful in detecting abnormal development. If the child fails two or more tests in the appropriate age group, he should be referred for further examination.

THE ASSESSMENT

History Taking

When an appointment is made for a paediatrician to see a probable handicapped child, an invitation should be sent, strongly recommending that *both* parents attend. A careful history obtained from the parents is the first essential.

Before the paediatrician talks to the parents, the child should be observed for a short time, fully dressed, with them. In many cases this gives the paediatrician some idea of the type of handicap and its extent, and will colour the questions he asks.

During the interview the child should sit on a parent's lap or play nearby. The talk with the parents should be friendly and relaxed. This attitude will affect the child, who will sense that they are talking to a friend and will himself be more disposed to be friendly and cooperative.

The following information must be obtained, but it need not be obtained in strict order. Often the parents will want to talk first of their worries about the child and his delayed milestones. These can then be filled in, and details of the family and the birth may be entered later on in the interview.

The Family

The parents must be asked about any significant illnesses or abnormalities in the family, and certain conditions can be specifically mentioned in a varied order: cleft palate, defective heart, fits, club foot, inability to walk, or mental backwardness. This will start a conversation about members of both sides of the family. Usually parents of a handicapped child will have discussed abnormalities in their families and a few questions will elucidate the nature of these illnesses.

At this stage, it is possible to draw a simple family tree. Details of siblings and their ages, and any miscarriages or still births can be recorded. It is, then, possible to go back at least two generations and hear about the child's uncles, aunts, cousins and grandparents. Any significant illness in the family must be given an accurate diagnosis if genetic advice is to make any sense and such information can be obtained from other doctors. Consanguinity in parents should be noted.

Pregnancy

The mother of a handicapped child will usually be more anxious to discuss her pregnancy than the mother of a non-handicapped child. Accidents, drug-taking, X-rays, threatened miscarriages, infection, pre-eclampsia and other illnesses must be recorded. Abnormalities, such as abnormal size and growth of the pregnancy, and absence of movements, may have significance.

Birth

The length of the pregnancy can usually be obtained from the mother. She will remember the expected date of birth, and prematurity or postmaturity by dates can be established. She will usually be accurate about the birth weight and the type of birth: forceps, breech or Caesarian. Many mothers will not know the reason for interfering with the normal process of birth. These details must be obtained from the maternity hospital. It is important to know whether the condition of the mother or the child caused concern.

Neonatal Period

As many children nowadays are born in hospital, and those who cause the mildest concern may be transferred to a special care unit, these details must be obtained from the maternity records. It has been found that a mother has not appreciated her child caused serious concern in the neonatal period, and vice versa. For accuracy in future research these findings must be checked. It is important to know the Apgar score; and if there were neonatal convulsions or twitchings, undue hypotonia, hypocalcaemia, hypoglycaemia or neonatal jaundice.

Problems in Infancy

The parents will be questioned about early problems with feeding, sucking, swallowing and chewing, and whether weaning on to solid food went smoothly. It should be noted whether there were sleep problems and if the baby was miserable or unduly quiet.

Milestones

The parents must be asked the times of specific milestones. The ones suggested are given in table 2.2. Other milestones must be recorded after direct observation.

These questions will be sufficient to pinpoint the parents' worries; and answering, the parents will elaborate the child's problems. It will also give them an opportunity to mention a deterioration.

Table 2.2

Milestone	Normal Age (*Rough estimate*)
Smiled	6 weeks
Sucked thumb	Early months
Reached for toys	6 months
Started babbling	3–4 months
Rolled over	6–8 months
Sat alone on floor	6–9 months
Attempted to crawl	9–10 months
Fed with biscuit	8–10 months
Played pat-a-cake	10–12 months
Walked alone	10–18 months
Said six single words	15–24 months
Fed with spoon	12–18 months
Walked upstairs alone	24–30 months
Said two word sentences	24 months
Recognised pictures	24–30 months
Scribbled	24–30 months
Asked questions	30–36 months
Said 'I' not 'me'	36 months
Took off shoes, socks, hat	18 months
Evidence of imaginative play	18 months onwards
Played with other children	36 months
Toilet training	Dry during day 2 years
	Night 3 years
	Bowel control 18 months

Illness and Immunisations

These must be documented. All visits to hospital, whether as outpatient or inpatient, should be checked. A direct question must be asked as to whether the child has had convulsions or a fit. If so, they must be accurately described.

Present Placement

We want to know if the child goes to a play group, or a normal or special school. This can be revealing, as it indicates the amount of concern the parents and the school authorities have already shown. Any separation from the parents should be recorded. The parents should have a chance to talk about their other children. This will highlight the abnormal development of the child, and give some insight into the parents' attitude to child rearing.

Occasionally it may be impossible to get a history direct from the parents. In these cases it is justifiable to get one with the help of a health visitor or social worker, who can visit the home. She might be given a form with the appropriate questions to answer.

EXAMINATION

Developmental Examination

The first part of the examination should be done with the child dressed. If he is a baby he will sit on his mother's lap. If he is an older infant, it is easier if this examination takes place with mother, child and examiner all sitting comfortably on a rug on the floor. If he is an older child, a well-fitting chair and table are needed.

There have been several studies on the development of normal children. Gesell (1947), Griffiths (1954), Sheridan (1960) and Illingworth (1971) have given us detailed notes which can be followed. Mary Sheridan's pamphlet, *The Developmental Progress of Infants and Young Children*, which can be obtained from Her Majesty's Stationery Office, is an ideal booklet for any paediatrician to carry around. Her notes are in no way an intelligence test, but they show what a child should be doing at a certain age, if he is functioning like his peers. They help the examiner to pinpoint delayed development in the four spheres: posture and large movements, vision and fine movements, hearing and speech, social behaviour and play. The examiner can either directly observe the child, or ask the mother questions, to see how he functions at each level according to these notes.

For a short developmental assessment taken from several observers, the form shown on page 6 has been very useful.

Apart from specific testing, which can be a lengthy process in a first examination, many paediatricians have their own base-lines of normal behaviour from which to assess an abnormality.

It is often a good idea at this stage to take the child from the mother and get the feel of him on one's own lap. Many parents are subconsciously ashamed of having a handicapped child, and have sensed the reluctance of relatives and friends to handle and cuddle him. If the paediatrician picks him up and plays with him, the parents realise the child is being considered a worthwhile person in his own right, and they will warm to the examination. The child should be held facing his mother so that he does not feel that he has lost her.

At the same time the paediatrician learns a lot from the feel of the child. He can assess head control, rigidity, balance, the way the child uses his hands, if he looks round to his mother, if he listens when she calls, if he grabs objects like the examiner's glasses (8–10 months level). The paediatrician will learn that a 6-month-old baby will come readily to someone else; but a 9-month-old baby starts to cry. This gives a crude idea that however handicapped the child, he may have normal intelligence. If he makes no objection one has reason to worry. With experience, this early handling of the child and simple play with toys can tell the paediatrician a great deal about him.

The child is then handed back to the parents, and the structured clinical examination takes place.

Testing of Hearing

For a baby up to the age of 18 months, the examiner relies on simple tests which show that the child can hear near at hand, quiet, everyday sounds. The clinical room should if possible be sound-deadened, and the examination should not take place if there are extraneous noises such as traffic passing. The child must not be tired or hungry. The sound must be made once only, five degrees behind the ear on both sides, so that the child cannot see the source of the sound. The sound must not cause a blowing or vibratory sensation which the child may feel rather than hear. The young child will not turn to a sound if it is made immediately behind the back of his head.

At 6 months of age the sound should be eighteen inches from the child's ear. The sounds used are the quiet rustle of toilet paper, a light bang of a spoon on the rim of a cup, rattles of different pitches, and the voice sounds of 'ps', 'ph', 'th' and 'oo'. The child should turn instantaneously to the sound, or momentarily stop what he is doing. Another observer should be present to verify his responses. For further verification the radio can be switched on suddenly though quietly behind the child, or somebody can speak unexpectedly though again quietly to him.

When small babies are being tested, the observations made by Murphy (1964) are helpful. He has recorded the ages and the manner in which small children turn to sound, and has also tabulated the ages at which babies develop the ability to make sounds, first vowels only, then dadda, mamma, and later 'g' and 'n'. The delay in normal response to sounds or in the start of normal babbling may be due to hearing loss, but it may be caused by mental backwardness or an inability to turn the head or the eyes. The mother's own observations must be taken into account.

For additional help, an appliance such as a Peters free-field audiometer may be used. This gives sounds of a known frequency at a calibrated intensity, and if the child will cooperate, it is possible to say that he hears a sound of a known intensity at a certain distance.

The child's response to speech may be noted by a person giving a quiet command like 'Give me the doll' or asking a question such as 'Would you like a sweetie?' behind him and watching his reaction.

For an older child a set of pictures can be used (Reed 1960). Each ear in turn is blocked with a finger. The child is asked in a quiet voice, 'Show me the ship' etc. The pictures have been chosen to test the child's hearing for normal speech, as well as to spot if he can hear the high frequency sounds 's', 'sh'. If the child can point quickly to all pictures when requested in a quiet voice ten feet away, there is no need to worry about hearing loss.

With these simple tests, which take only a few minutes, an estimate can be made as to whether we need to worry about the child's hearing; and they can be carried out on one who is fairly severely handicapped. If there is slight worry, the child should be referred for full audiological assessment (as described in chapter 4) using methods such as observations through a one-way screen, conditioning and evoked response audiometry.

Testing of Vision

As Sheridan (1960) has shown, a 1-month-old baby turns his head towards the light, and follows a pencil flash lamp with his eyes at a distance of one foot. By the age of 6 months he is 'visually insatiable', and moves his head and eyes eagerly in every direction.

If a handicapped child takes no interest visually in his surroundings, we must decide whether this is due to an inability to move his head or eyes, to mental backwardness or defective vision.

Reaction of the pupils to sudden light gives some idea if there is sight. A sluggish or inactive pupil is always pathological.

Tests of sight in the early months are largely subjective. The parents and examiner will notice what the child appears to see—a large doll or his dinner.

By 6–8 months he can be tested with white rolling balls as described by Sheridan (1960). At 6 months a baby will watch a white rolling ball of two inch, one inch, or half inch diameter at a distance of ten feet, and by 9 months a ball of a quarter inch diameter at the same distance. These tests indicate adequate vision. By 18 months he can be tested on the miniature toys in the Stycar vision test at ten feet. He will match a small toy with one of the same shape but different colour in a set which is shown to him. At $2\frac{1}{2}$–3 years he can match the letters V, O, T, H, at ten feet; and from that age a definite idea of his visual acuity can be made. Near vision can be tested by letters in a similar way.

The child may also have a field of vision defect. This can be tested by confrontation methods or by watching the child's eye movement through a horizontal slit in a vertical board, and seeing when he notices small balls on a stick as they are brought into his line of vision. Tunnel vision and serious defects can be detected in very handicapped children.

With a mentally handicapped child, the problem may be more complicated. A mongol of 6 years may only just manage the Stycar letter test, and may only just achieve the toy matching test. If he is myopic this is too late to find out. Severely handicapped cerebral palsied children may have difficulty in sitting up, and limitation of eye movements and head turning may make the tests difficult to perform.

Possibly all handicapped children should see an ophthalmologist. There may be optic atrophy, retinal defects, cataracts, astigmatism, as well as refractive errors, and eye movement and field of vision defects. This is true of deaf, mentally handicapped, cerebral palsied children, children with spina bifida, and children with handicaps such as educational subnormality. The fundi, lens, media and retina may be examined after dilation with a mydriatic; more difficult cases may call for an eye examination under anaesthesia or a visual response electroencephalogram.

Only developmental tests should be attempted at the first examination; fuller ophthalmological examination should be deferred until later.

CLINICAL EXAMINATION

The child must now be undressed; but if the early play and developmental examination has been pleasant, he will be willing to cooperate. The type of examination is influenced by the history and the observations already made.

The child's weight and height should be measured, and compared with percentile curves.

The head circumference, width and length must be measured, and compared with recognised scales (table 2.3).

The head shape, slant of eyes, position and formation of ears, abnormalities of nose, lip and chin, and other evidence of an abnormal face must be described in writing. Abnormal body measurements must be recorded, as must defects of skin, limbs, spine, sacrum, hips and genital organs. The heart should be examined for congenital defect. All this will take only a short time.

A preliminary study of movement defects must decide whether they are primarily due to a central nervous system defect as in cerebral palsy, a spinal cord abnormality as in spina bifida, or muscle disease as in muscular dystrophy.

Table 2.3 Head circumference for boys and girls during the first seven years of life (after Westropp & Barber, *Growth of the Skull in Young Children*, Oxford)

	Boys	Girls
Age	Mean (cm)	Mean (cm)
1 month	37·3	36·5
3 month	40·7	39·8
6 month	43·6	42·5
9 month	45·7	44·6
1 year	46·8	45·6
1½ year	47·9	47·0
2 year	49·1	48·0
2½ year	49·8	48·8
3 year	50·4	49·5
3½ year	51·0	50·1
4 year	51·2	50·7
4½ year	51·6	51·0
5 year	51·8	51·2
7 year	52·7	52·2

NEUROLOGICAL EXAMINATION

In any child with suspected brain pathology, this examination is of prime importance. It has less definitive emphasis than in the adult. If the child's brain has developed abnormally or been damaged early in life, there will be alteration in the development and disappearance of primitive reflexes. It is essential therefore to have a knowledge of normal infantile reflexes and their time of disappearance, and table 2.4 gives guidance on these matters.

Bobath (1956), Paine and Oppé (1966), Milani (1967) and Illingworth (1971) have shown how these reflexes affect the normal movement patterns; and how an abnormal reflex pattern prevents the development of normal movements.

Paine and Oppé state 'These signs may be more helpful than conventional neurological signs based on alterations of muscle tone, reflexes etc.'

The cranial nerves should be examined, as damage to a cranial nerve such as the third, sixth or seventh may be present. Evidence of hypertonia or hypotonia in muscle groups in different postures, and normal reflexes such as the knee-jerk and plantar response, should be recorded.

Factors which must be recorded are:

Head control in prone and supine positions.

Eye movement patterns, strabismus, incoordination of movement and inability to move the eyes in any direction.

Difficulties in swallowing or chewing, and evidence of excessive dribbling. Any motor-speech problems.

Ability to roll over, whether in a total extensor pattern using the head as a lever, or smoothly with alternative flexion and extension of the head, body and legs.

Ability to sit up. Whether the curve of the back is normal, or the child shows the infantile curve.

Whether he can save himself by outward thrust of the arms if pushed over.

Position of the arms when lying supine. Whether he lies in full extension with arms retracted at the shoulders, or if he can bring them to his side.

What he does if held prone and suddenly tilted forwards.

Position of the child on all fours kneeling.

Whether he holds himself with arms extended and hips partially flexed. What happens when his head is flexed or extended.

Whether he can crawl smoothly or makes bunny hops.

Can he save himself if pushed over?

Can he bring either hand to his mouth to suck?

Can he approximate both hands in the sitting position?

Can he pronate and supinate his forearms?

Description of his hand grasp: whether a whole hand grasp, an ulnar grasp, a thumb and fingers grasp, or a pincer movement of thumb and finger.

Does he show an avoiding or a grasping reaction in his hands?

His posture when held erect: whether adduction and internal rotation of the hips, extension of the legs and plantar flexion; or abduction and eversion of feet.

Can he stand and balance in standing?

Is there ankle clonus?

Can his ankles be dorsiflexed with knees straight?

Description of his gait.

Table 2.4

Reflex	Description	Timing
Moro reflex	The baby is placed supine and the back of the head is supported on the palm of the hand, an inch above the table. Rapid release of the hand causes abduction and extension of the arms, with partial opening of the hand. This is often followed by adduction of the arms and crying.	Present from birth to 4 months
Placing	The anterior aspect of the leg or arm is brought against the edge of a table. The child lifts the leg up to step on to the table, or elevates the arms to place the hand on the table.	From birth onwards
Stepping reflex	The baby is held erect on a table with the sole of the foot pressed against it. This initiates a few steps of reciprocal walking.	From birth to 4 weeks
Positive supporting	When the sole of the foot is pressed on the table, the legs and body straighten in a standing posture.	Birth to 2 months. Then absent till 6 months. Reappears when foot grasp goes
Hand grasp	An object, possibly the examiner's finger, is placed in the baby's palm from the ulnar side. The baby's fingers grip tightly.	Birth to 3 months. Disappears when hand can be used for support
Foot grasp	The grasp is elicited by stroking the sole of the foot behind the toes.	Birth to 8 months when foot can be used for support
Asymmetrical tonic neck reflex	The head is rotated to either side with the shoulders horizontal. The arm and leg towards which the head is rotated extend and the other arm and leg flex.	Present 1–4 months, but never strong. Prevents rolling and the hand feeling the face

Table 2.4—*Continued*

Symmetrical tonic neck reflex	With the child on all fours, the neck is extended, there is marked extension of the arms and flexing of the hips and lower limbs. When the neck is flexed, the lower limbs extend.	Appears briefly at 6–8 months at first crawl
Labyrinth tonic reflex	The child shows increased exterior tone when lying supine, and increased flexor tone when lying prone.	Tendency shown only feebly at birth
Landau reflex	If the child is held in ventral suspension, the head, spine and legs extend.	From 3–6 months. Disappears at 12 months
Righting reflex	When the child is pulled up by the hands, the head is raised to be level with the body.	From birth to 4 months
Neck-righting reflex	Turning the head to one side is followed by movement of the body as a whole.	From birth. Strong at 3 months
Body-righting reflex on body	Modifies the child's early attempt to rise and stand. Child struggles if supine.	7–12 months
Balance reactions in sitting	When the child is in the sitting posture and is pushed over, the arm extends laterally to prevent falling.	4–9 months. Must be present before safe sitting
Balance reactions in standing or tiltive reactions	When the standing child is pushed laterally, his leg and hand extend to prevent falling.	5–12 months. Must be present before standing is possible
Parachute reaction	The child is held round the waist and lowered head downwards toward a table. He extends his arms and hands to save himself.	From 6 months. Present throughout life

The last six reflexes remain throughout life.

Crude sensation and stereognosis may be tested by placing objects such as a marble, penny or safety pin in the child's hand without his looking, and asking him to name the objects. If he will not speak, he can point to the appropriate object in a second set placed on a table. Children of 3 years will cooperate in this way.

A description should be written of exactly what the child can do and how he does it. A photograph or film is of value. The child's difficulties may defy description in neurological terms since these are often a mixture of primitive reflexes which have not disappeared, delayed balance reactions, abnormal muscle tone, perhaps early contractures or sensory loss, visual defect or defective body image. But shining through these difficulties may be the child's voluntary attempt to overcome his handicaps.

Advice

After this first prolonged examination, the paediatrician will be in a position to have a preliminary chat with the parents about the child's condition and programme of treatment; but it must be stressed that further examinations are necessary.

FURTHER EXAMINATIONS

As a routine, all handicapped children should have a full range of scientific investigations. These should include X-ray of skull and wrist for bone age, tests for aminoaciduria, electroencephalogram, chromosome investigations (in the majority of cases), biochemical estimations (calcium, phosphorus, alkaline phosphatase), blood lead estimation and blood uric acid (in some cases). Antibody titre estimations for rubella, toxoplasmosis and cytomegalic virus disease may be indicated.

PSYCHOLOGICAL EXAMINATION

It should be stressed that all handicapped children should be seen by a psychologist. His aim is not to obtain a numerical intelligence quotient or a firm prediction about the child's educational future, but to analyse his abilities and difficulties in all cognitive and learning fields, and to pass on this information to those people dealing with the care of the child—doctor, teachers, therapists and often educational administrators.

Associated Professional Opinions

Soon after the clinical examination, a handicapped child will be seen by the physiotherapist, speech therapist and occupational therapist. Each will assess him in a different light and their early descriptions of what he can do will form a basis for treatment. A social worker should visit the home and report back to the team.

Assessment Centre

This means that for the full assessment of a handicapped child, two or three prolonged visits to a clinic are required. They should be made as easy as possible, and transport if necessary supplied. Ideally they should take place in a purpose-built assessment centre.

After the assessment, and possibly after a case conference on the child, both parents must be seen again by the paediatrician to discuss the whole problem. It is best if these assessments can be made with the child as an outpatient, but if admission is necessary, the mother should be admitted with the child. The place of residence, if possible, should have hostel-type provision rather than a hospital bed.

REFERENCES

BOBATH K & BOBATH B (1956) The diagnosis of cerebral palsy in infancy. *Arch. Dis. Childh.* **31**, 408.
EGAN D F, ILLINGWORTH R S & MACKEITH R C (1969) *Developmental Screens 0–5 years. Clinics in Developmental Medicine*, No. 30. Spastics Society & William Heinemann, London
GESELL A & AMATRUDA C S (1947) *Developmental Diagnosis.* Hoeber, New York
GRIFFITHS R (1954) *The Abilities of Babies.* University of London Press, London
ILLINGWORTH R S (1971) *The Development of the Infant and Young Child.* E & S Livingstone, London
MILANI COMPARETTI A & GIDONI E A (1967) Routine developmental examination in normal and retarded children. *Dev. Med. Childh. Neurol.* **9**, 631
MURPHY K (1964) Development of normal vocalisation and speech. *The Child Who does not Talk. Clinics in Developmental Medicine*, No. 13. Spastics Society & William Heinemann, London

PAINE R S & OPPÉ T (1966) *Neurological Examination of Children. Clinics in Developmental Medicine*, 20/21. Spastics Society & William Heinemann, London

PARFITT J (1971) *Physical and Mental Assessment.* National Children's Bureau, London

ROSENBLOOM L & HORTON M E (1971) The maturation of fine prehension in young children. *Dev. Med. Childh. Neurol.* **13**, 3

SHERIDAN M (1960) Vision screening of very young or handicapped children. *Brit. med. J.* **2**, 453

SHERIDAN M (1962) Infants at risk of handicapping conditions. *Monthly Bulletin, Ministry of Health Laboratory Service* **21**, 238

SHERIDAN M (1968) *The Developmental Progress of Infants and Young Children.* Department of Health and Social Security, Report No. 102. HMSO, London

Chapter 3
The Child with a Severe Hearing Loss

In discussing a 'deaf child' or, more exactly, a child with a hearing loss, we must first define his handicap. Hearing is necessary for the comprehension of speech; it is the reception of sound by the ear, and its transmission to the auditory area of the cortex. To hear normally, the entire auditory apparatus of the child must be functioning. Sound must be able to pass along the external auditory meatus and impinge on the drum. The transmission of sounds through the middle ear by the ossicles must be adequate. From the middle ear, the sound waves must pass via the oval window to the cochlea and the organ of Corti. From there, the sensations are translated into nerve pulses and pass via the lateral and ventral cochlei nuclei to the olives, and then to the medial geniculate body and the temporal lobe of the cortex. From these nerve pathways there are other connections to ear, eye and body muscles, and other parts of the cortex.

If the defect in hearing is due to an abnormality of the outer or middle ear, it is called a *conductive* hearing loss. If it is due to abnormality of the cochlea or the organs of Corti, or of any part of the auditory nerve pathways, it is called a *perceptive* hearing loss.

Measurement

Sounds reach the ears at a speed of 760 miles per hour. Each pure sound has a particular wave pattern which is called its frequency. Frequency is measured in number of cycles per second or *Hertz* (Hz). Middle C is 256 Hz. The range of the normal voice is 200–4000 Hz. The higher frequency sounds include the 's', 'sh', etc. of normal speech. It is said that a normal ear can detect sounds of frequency 20–30,000 Hz.

The intensity or loudness of a sound is measured in *decibels* (dB). For the student of physics it must be stated that this measurement of the intensity of sound is not a pure arithmetical one. A sound of 60 dB is not twice as loud as a sound of 30 dB. The number is a ratio only and the figures given are based on a logarithmic unit. The lowest sound that can be heard has an intensity of 10–16 watts. A bel is a logarithmic unit to the base 10 of the ratio between the given intensity and this lowest sound. A decibel is 1/10 of a bel. This prevents very large numbers being used. A quiet whisper has an intensity of about 30 dB, a conversational voice 60 dB and a loud shout 90 dB. In an ordinary conversation the loudness of different words or syllables may vary as much as 30 dB. In testing adults and older children for suspected hearing loss, one needs to obtain an exact audiogram from both ears. Three types of audiogram are shown in figure 3.1.

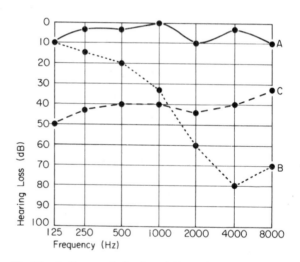

Fig. 3.1 Audiograms indicating: A Normal hearing
B High frequency hearing loss
C Moderate hearing loss

Conductive Hearing Loss

In the case of a conductive hearing loss, the audiogram shows an even loss of hearing in all frequencies. The nerve pathways and inner ear are intact, and sounds can bypass the middle ear and reach the auditory nerve by bone conduction through the temporal bone. A person with a conductive hearing loss will hear better by bone conduction than by air conduction. A tuning fork is placed near the affected ear, and the child informs the examiner when he no longer hears the sound. The tuning fork is immediately placed on the mastoid process of that ear. If a conductive hearing loss is present the child will then signify that he can again hear the sound. These tests can only be made on an older cooperative child.

Perceptive Hearing Loss

When there is a perceptive hearing loss, the audiogram shows an uneven loss of hearing in different frequencies. Often the hearing for high frequency sounds is more selectively damaged. This is presumably due to a selective lack of development or damage of parts of the cochlea or the cochlear nuclei. Amplification by a hearing aid can cause distortion of sounds. In perceptive or 'nerve deafness', a phenomenon called *recruitment* may occur. After a certain amplification, sounds in the affected ear may become painfully loud and, if both ears are affected, may appear louder in the one which is worse affected. This effect may be very unpleasant, and may cause an adult or child to refuse to wear a hearing aid.

Types of Hearing Loss

The hearing loss is rarely *total*.

It may be so severe as to be called *subtotal*.

In the majority of cases, the loss may be only *partial*, and as already mentioned may involve the *high frequency* tones solely or more markedly.

A hearing loss may be *unilateral*.

In cases of what is called *central deafness* or *central communication disorder* it can be shown that the child hears but cannot translate what he hears into meaning, either the meaning of language or the significance of everyday sounds. This is discussed in chapter 14.

We must also know if the child was born deaf or if he acquired deafness after a period of understanding language, but before speech developed. The overall effect of a severe hearing loss is affected by the child's intelligence and by the presence of additional handicaps.

Referral

The child will be referred to a paediatrician or an otologist because a hearing loss is suspected. In many cases the mother will have suspected a hearing loss, and this should always be considered grounds for referral. Simple tests for hearing in an 'infant welfare' or 'well baby' clinic may have suggested a defect. The child's name may be on an 'at risk' register. There may be a particular likelihood of deafness, as in cases of maternal rubella or neonatal jaundice.

Other indications of a possible hearing loss are when:
a the child babbles at the normal time, and then ceases to babble;
b language is not developing;
c the child is avidly watching adults with his eyes, and turning to look more than usual;
d he understands simple commands when gesture is used, but cannot understand double commands.

The child should be fully assessed in a well-planned audiology department.

History Taking

The history should be as thorough as that for any paediatric examination. The family history and any antenatal, perinatal and postnatal abnormalities should be recorded. Information about all significant illnesses, e.g. rubella in pregnancy, must specifically be asked for. The taking of drugs in pregnancy, quinine, streptomycin, neomycin, kanamycin or salicylates, must be noted. Questions must be asked about childish illnesses, the infectious fevers, upper respiratory infections, particularly ear infections, and any significant accidents.

The mother should be asked about the baby's early reactions to sound, whether he babbled, if he has stopped babbling, the types of sounds he makes, whether he is understanding speech, if he speaks, and if his speech is distorted.

A deaf child will babble in the early months of life, but when he gets no feedback from his babbling, as he cannot hear it or enjoy it, the babbling will cease. He may go on to use the 'm' and 'd', which are the first consonants used by hearing children at about 6 months, but will not go on to use the sounds 'p', 'b', 't', 'n', which babies use in their babble at about 8–9 months. He will not copy adult speech with the rhythmic intonation of a normal baby of 6–8 months.

Audiology Unit

It is hoped that the testing of hearing can take place in a well-planned and, if possible, purpose-built audiology unit, where there are full facilities for paediatric, audiological and psychological assessment, and the services on the premises of appropriate technicians and of a teacher of the deaf.

The room in which the child is tested should be sound-deadened. Ideally the walls should be nine inches thick and lined with sound-absorbent tiles. There should be double doors, double glazing on the windows and a carpet on the floor. One wall should be fitted with a one-way screen for observation. The room should not be less than ten feet by six feet. There should be a tape recording machine outside the room which can feed sounds into two loudspeakers at different corners of the room. The room itself should be gay and pleasant, and have suitable toys and pictures. Other apparatus such as the Stycar hearing test material, a free-field audiometer, an audiometer and a speech audiometer should be available; and a sound-level meter, a machine to calibrate the sounds used for testing. The room can be fitted with one microphone or more, so that the child's babble in any part of the room can be heard in the adjoining one.

The person testing hearing should have a special interest in hearing assessment, and also a good knowledge of normal child development and play.

TESTS FOR HEARING

The methods used for testing will vary according to the child's age.

Orientation Reflex

In the neonatal period the newborn baby should respond to sound close to his ear by a modified Moro response or even merely an eye blink. It is possible to be certain that a baby of this age reacts at least by reflex to sound of different intensities.

Distraction Technique

These methods can be used from early babyhood to $2-2\frac{1}{2}$ years. While being tested the child should be playing with a toy so that, with this distraction, he will not tend to turn round and watch what the examiner is doing. The examiner makes the sound five degrees behind the level of the ear, and eighteen inches from each ear. A second examiner should sit in front of the child and watch his reaction.

The sounds used for testing may be loud: a drum, xylophone, or squeaky toy, which have an intensity of about 75 decibels. Quieter sounds of the level of 40–60 decibels, such as the rustle of paper or the clink of a spoon on the rim of a cup, should then be used. The testing is completed by using quiet voice sounds.

The baby reacts by turning round, or by a slight twitch or eye blink. He may momentarily cease crying, or there may be a sudden stilling of his play; and this gives a definite clue that he has heard the sound. The baby of 3–6 months will often respond once only. Generally, from 6–8 months of age, he will turn to a familiar sound instantaneously, and if he hears the voice, will copy the intonation. From 9–14 months he will turn in any direction to a sound that interests him. It must be remembered that there are normal children who do not follow these rules, and confound the examiner by taking no notice of what he is doing.

From 14–24 months he should respond to speech sounds and simple requests, and show an interest in the speech he is hearing. From 2–3 years the child can be tested by specific demands, as in the Stycar hearing tests. All these sounds can be calibrated in a free field.

For a child under 3 years it should be possible to report positive findings, for example, that he can hear a sound of such a frequency at an intensity of so many decibels at so many feet; and a report can be given on his response to speech. From these findings it should be possible to decide whether the child has a serious hearing loss, and if special help is needed, such as from a hearing aid or from a teacher of the preschool deaf.

Conditioning Technique

From about the age of 3 years, it should be possible to obtain a fairly exact audiogram from each ear. Over a period of several sessions with a therapist or audiologist the child is taught to make a certain action whenever he hears a sound. The action may be putting a brick in a cup, or some even simpler action, such as knocking a brick off the table. When he understands what he must do, and the situation has developed into a constructive game, he is tested with an earphone on each ear in turn. If he is cooperative it is possible to obtain an audiogram. His response to sounds in each frequency, and in each intensity, can be recorded. With patience, and after several sessions in the audiology clinic, success can be obtained in most children of normal intelligence, even if they are physically handicapped, as in the case of cerebral palsied children. If the child will not tolerate earphones a free-field audiometer can be used (figure 3.2).

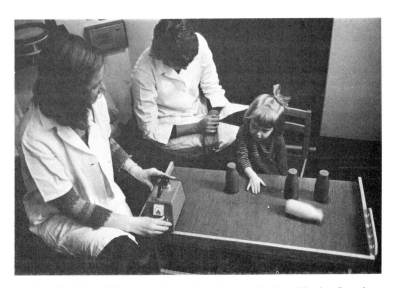

Fig. 3.2   The child's hearing is tested by the method of conditioning. Sounds of varying pitch and intensity are emitted from the Peter's free-field audiometer. The child knocks down a toy when she can hear the sound.

Response to Speech Sounds

The young child's response to speech can be tested by the Rhyming word picture test (Reed 1960) or the Stycar hearing test with toys and pictures (Sheridan 1968). A page of pictures of objects such as fish, ship, seat, pig is put in front of the child and he is asked to point to the object spoken at varying degrees of loudness and distance from each ear. When the child is older a speech audiogram can be obtained. A list of phonetically balanced words, i.e. words that contain all the vowels and consonants of normal speech, is played to the child from a tape recorder at a known intensity of sound. Either in free field, or wearing an earphone, he repeats the words he hears. A speech audiogram is a graph where the percentage of words heard is plotted against the amplification in decibels.

Evoked Response Audiometry

To make a diagnosis with a child who is either severely handicapped physically or mentally, or withdrawn and uncooperative, an apparatus such as an evoked response audiometer can be used. This test is based on the fact that a sound, if heard, will make an appreciable change in the electroencephalogram. The sounds are repeated twenty to thirty times, and an inbuilt computer gives an average measure of the increased amplitude of the brain waves when sounds are heard. By this method it is possible to detect which sounds the child is hearing in each ear, and to get a threshold when he can only just hear the sound. A result can be obtained which is accurate within 20 decibels. It is useful for the most severely handicapped, the autistic and the very young child, where it is important to know if there is a hearing loss. The accuracy of this method in children has been doubted particularly if the child has an intermittent abnormal brain wave pattern. The child must usually be sedated.

Electrocochleography

Children tested by electrocochleography must be anaesthetised and a 0·3 mm electrode is inserted through the ear drum to rest on the promontory of the middle ear, near the basal coil of the cochlea. The response of the cochlea to different sounds at different frequencies is recorded electrically. This gives a record of the child's hearing as it involves the cochlea and the auditory nerve pathways up to, but not including, the cortex.

Crossed Acoustic Response

This method, described by Douek et al, records the postauricular muscle response to hearing. Electrodes are placed behind the ear and the response to sounds passed through the ear phones to either ear is recorded. This tests the response of the cochlea, the cochlea nucleus and the nerve pathways across the brain stem to sound.

Autism and Mental Handicap

A distinction must be made between hearing loss and mental backwardness. A young mentally handicapped child may not respond to any stimuli. This can be tested by noting his response to a puff of air or a bright light. If he reacts quickly to these stimuli, but not to sound, there is a strong suspicion of deafness.

The differential diagnosis between a severe hearing loss and autism may be difficult, particularly if the child has not learnt to lip read, and takes no notice of adults' faces. By careful observation in a sound deadened room the autistic child can be shown to take notice of quiet sounds occasionally. In difficult cases the child can be tested by electrical methods.

Impedance Test in Audiometry

This is a test of middle ear function in cases of suspected conductive hearing loss. Soundwaves of different frequencies are impinged on the ear drum, and the wave reflected off the drum is measured. A tense or a flaccid drum can be diagnosed. Fluid or a negative pressure in the middle ear can be detected, as well as tympanitic or ossicular rigidity. If the reaction after swallowing is tested, patency of the Eustachian tube can be ascertained.

DIAGNOSIS OF
CAUSE OF DEAFNESS

If, after careful audiometric testing, a diagnosis of deafness is made, the paediatrician or otologist should try to ascertain the aetiology.

The causes of childhood deafness are:

CONDUCTIVE DEAFNESS
> Congenital abnormalities of outer ear
> Wax
> Foreign body
> Chronic otitis media (and upper
> respiratory infection)
> Glue ear

Congenital abnormalities of middle ear
In association with cleft palate
Head injury
Treacher Collins' syndrome
   (mandibulofacial dysostosis)
Crouzon's disease
   (craniofacial dysostosis)
Thalidomide taken in pregnancy
Associated recessive renal, genital
   and middle ear abnormalities

PERCEPTIVE DEAFNESS

Inherited
Dominant deafness (pure form)
Recessive deafness (pure form)
Down's syndrome
Hurler's (gargoylism) syndrome
Pendred's syndrome
Waardenburg syndrome
In association with other syndromes,
   Klipper-Feil, albinism, Refsum's syndrome
In association with nephritis (Alport's disease)
Deafness with abnormal heart condition
   (Fraser 1964)
Forms of retinitis pigmentosa
   (Usher's syndrome)

Prenatal
Maternal influenza
Maternal rubella
Maternal syphilis
Streptomycin, neomycin, kanamycin, quinine,
   salicylates, taken in pregnancy

Perinatal
Prematurity

Neonatal
Asphyxia
Jaundice

Postnatal
Meningitis—various infective agents
Encephalitis
Measles
Pertussis
Dihydroxystreptomycin treatment for
   meningitis or other infection
Head injury

Conductive Deafness

This is due to abnormalities of the external or middle ear. Wax or a foreign body may cause a partial hearing loss, and will be seen on auroscopic examination.

Abnormalities of the External Ear

Atresia of the external auditory meatus may occur. The atresia may be complete or there may be a blind pocket. A small pinna (microtia) or accessory auricles or a congenital fistula in front of the helix may be present. As the outer and middle ears develop from the first branchial arch, and the inner ear from the plaque of external ectoderm and mesoderm, which becomes differentiated to form the cochlea and semicircular canals, it is unlikely that abnormalities of the inner and middle ear will both be present. This means that in cases of abnormalities of the middle ear, the cochlea and auditory pathways may be intact. Children with an abnormal external auditory meatus should have surgery to open up the canal. The age of 18 months is thought to be the optimum time for surgery, and at this age it is possible to obtain an X-ray to verify the presence of the cochlea.

Abnormalities of the Middle Ear

Abnormalities of the middle ear and ossicles have been found to be the cause of deafness in some children whose mothers took the drug *thalidomide* in early pregnancy. Repair and reconstruction of the middle ear have improved hearing.

Infective Conditions

Severe deafness due to *chronic otitis media* should not be seen nowadays with the use of antibiotics. A few cases do occur, particularly from social class V. These cases should be seen regularly by an otologist, as operations such as tympanoplasty—repair of the drums—may help.

A recently noted condition called *glue ear* causes mild deafness today. The middle ear becomes filled with mucopurulent matter following inadequately treated middle ear infection with antibiotics.

The drum has not been perforated. This condition occurs more readily in handicapped children, who are more liable to get repeated upper respiratory infections. It has been noted particularly following maternal rubella. It can be serious in a blind child, who relies so much on his hearing.

Cleft Palate

This may be associated with deafness due to middle ear abnormality.

Head Injury

This is a rare cause of damage to the middle ear and ossicles.

Treacher Collins' Syndrome

In this syndrome there is a maldevelopment of the faciomaxillary area with high palate and crowding of the teeth. The pinnae are usually prominent, and the eyes have an antimongoloid slant. The accompanying deafness is due to maldevelopment of the middle ear and ossicles.

Perceptive Deafness

In this group of cases the damage or abnormality is in the cochlea or auditory nerve pathways. The causes are genetic, prenatal or perinatal in origin, or due to infection in later life.

Hereditary Causes

In any school for the partially hearing, there will be a number of children whose sole handicap is a hearing loss; and the presumed cause is a genetic one. Not infrequently one parent or both has also been born deaf. If the form of deafness in the parents is a dominant condition, the chances of a child being affected are as high as 50%. If the deafness in the parents is a recessive form, even if both are affected, the chances of the offspring being affected are lowered to 1 in 4 or 25%. Due to the enclosed life of deaf adults, and the fact that they meet each other in clubs for the hard of hearing, marriage among two born-deaf people is quite common, and this remains a source of candidates for schools for the deaf. As many of these deaf people are employed, happy and emotionally secure, there is a feeling among social workers for the deaf that these marriages should not be discouraged. A deaf child born into such a family learns to communicate with his parents, and is often a lively outgoing child. The hearing child of such a union is not necessarily maladjusted, and should be helped at an early age by attendance at a nursery school. About one-third of all cases of congenital deafness of this type, and presumably many of the 20–30% of cases where no cause can be found, are also cases of the recessive form of congenital deafness. The deafness in these cases is usually profound. Pathologically the organ of Corti and the saccule are represented by a mass of undifferentiated cells, and the sensory epithelium is of a fetal type.

Other forms of deafness due to inherited conditions and congenital abnormalities are associated with additional abnormalities, and fall into defined syndromes.

Down's Syndrome (mongolism) A fair proportion of these children have a congenital form of deafness. For this reason all of these children should have an early test for hearing. They can be helped as babies. In later childhood some will tolerate a hearing aid.

Hurler's Syndrome (gargoylism) (see page 183) The manifestations of this condition are short stature, short neck, a large dolicocephalic head with coarse hair, thick lips, thick low-set ears, hirsutism, lumbar lordosis, flexion contractures, claw-like hands, hepatosplenomegaly, cardiac defects, herniae, corneal clouding and partial hearing loss. These children are mentally retarded. The condition is due to an inborn error in mucopolysaccharide metabolism and there are various forms; Hunter's, Morquio Ullrich and Morquio Brailsford diseases. These children are easily recognised. It is important to test their hearing.

Pendred's Syndrome The children with this syndrome have a recessive form of deafness and in middle childhood develop an enlarged thyroid gland, which is usually euthyroid. The two conditions may be independent manifestations of the same recessive genetic defect.

Waardenburg Syndrome In this dominantly inherited syndrome a child shows asymmetric colouring of the irides, a white forelock and skin pigmentation, a lateral displacement of the medial canthi, and a broad nasal ridge, over which the eyebrows often meet. There is a perceptive deafness which may be partial. The loss may be in the middle frequencies and not in the high frequencies. The severe hearing loss may not be noted by teachers if the child is a good lip reader. Patients with this type of defect have been seen in hospitals for the subnormal, as the deafness has not been spotted.

A hearing loss may be a serious but secondary handicap associated with other recessive conditions.

Retinitis Pigmentosa There are several varieties of retinal abnormality (Fraser 1964) which are described under the overall heading of retinitis pigmentosa. The pigmentation in the retina and the retinal changes vary in different forms of the syndrome. Deafness is an associated handicap. Any child with defective sight due to this condition should have a careful test of hearing. Children with a genetic form of deafness should be examined ophthalmologically at intervals for the development of this condition. The first symptom may be night blindness in a child who already has a hearing loss. Some forms of this condition are associated with a vestibulocerebellar form of ataxia (Refsum's syndrome).

Prenatal

The condition which at the present time takes preeminence as the cause of deafness is *maternal rubella*, where the mother had 'german measles' in the first few months of pregnancy. In many centres a high proportion of the newly discovered cases of deafness in infants is due to this cause. These affected children are nearly always multiply handicapped. Cataracts, congenital heart defect and mental subnormality are often also present. There are occasional cases, more frequent in some epidemics than others, where deafness is the only manifestation. There is some evidence that if hearing alone is affected the time of the maternal rubella was late—in the third or fourth month of pregnancy. More severely affected children with eye defects followed an earlier infection. This condition will be further described under the 'deaf-blind' child.

Maternal Syphilis has been a cause of deafness commencing at 2–10 years in the past and is usually associated with other stigmata. The condition should not be forgotten, but cases should not occur with adequate antenatal care and treatment.

Other Infections, such as influenza in early pregnancy, and in particular the 'Asian' form, have been blamed for congenital deafness.

Cretinism and endemic goitre may be associated with deafness due to a defect in the organ of Corti.

Drugs taken during pregnancy can damage the baby's hearing. Quinine has been particularly blamed. It may have been taken as an antimalarial drug or as an abortifacient. Other toxic drugs are streptomycin, kanamycin, neomycin and salicylate.

Perinatal

Extreme prematurity may be the prime cause of deafness in some cases, usually due to neonatal jaundice, but severe maternal tox-aemia has been implicated. Neonatal asphyxia has been followed by deafness, usually of the high frequency type. Fisch (1969) has suggested that the anoxia may selectively damage the cochlear nuclei or render it more sensitive to damage by bilirubin.

Neonatal Jaundice

Jaundice in the neonatal period may be due to the inability of the liver to excrete conjugated bilirubin, but in some cases of deafness following premature birth, jaundice was due to excessive doses of vitamin K given to prevent haemorrhagic disease of the newborn (Laurence). These cases should no longer occur.

The most common cause of neonatal jaundice is haemolytic disease of the newborn, due to Rh or ABO isoimmunisation. Rise of rhesus antibodies antenatally should be detected, and repeated bilirubin estimations should be performed in the early neonatal period. Immediate exchange transfusions should be given if the serum bilirubin rises above 18 mg/ml. It is known, however, that hearing can be impaired by lower levels in cases of anoxia, particularly in premature babies. Other cases of neonatal jaundice are due to glucose-6-phosphate dehydrogenase or pyruvate kinase deficiencies. This occurs more commonly in the Chinese and Japanese races.

The type of deafness may be a high frequency loss only, which means that cases may go unnoticed. Alternatively the hearing loss may be severe, but more marked in the higher frequencies.

Postnatal

A hearing child may become severely deaf with a perceptive form of deafness following meningitis due to various organisms. Deafness may also follow a viral encephalitis. It has been particularly noticed after measles and mumps, where the condition was presumably an encephalitis. Streptomycin in the treatment of tuberculous meningitis was a cause in the past. These children who lose their hearing need immediate training and educational help to prevent them also losing the speech they have acquired.

Additional Handicaps

When we study the list of possible causes of childhood deafness it can be seen that in a large number of conditions the child is likely to have an additional handicap. In fact it is only in some cases of conductive hearing loss and in the hereditary forms of pure deafness that an additional handicap is not a feature. Defects of sight are likely to occur, particularly in the postrubella syndrome, retinitis pigmentosa, and all cases where there is brain pathology. This means that in cases of hearing loss vision should be carefully assessed.

Associated congenital defects may occur in all the inherited and prenatal conditions. Cerebral palsy, a defect of movement due to brain damage, may occur. Following neonatal jaundice, athetosis due to kernicterus is as common as the high frequency hearing loss; and the two conditions are frequently coexistent. The child may have a mild high frequency loss and severe athetosis, or a severe hearing loss and very minor evidence of athetosis, or one of the many combinations in between. Deafness may follow a premature birth or perinatal anoxia, and both these can also cause spastic cerebral palsy of various types.

A hearing defect of any type may be associated with mental defect of severely subnormal (IQ under 50) or educationally subnormal (IQ 50–75) levels.

Differential Diagnosis

In cases of mental subnormality a hearing loss may be missed, especially if it is a partial loss. Similarly children with a hearing loss are in serious danger of being considered mentally or educationally subnormal.

For instance, it was found that a bright-eyed, superficially intelligent little boy of seven years was unable to carry out a double command, such as 'Give this to Mrs Brown and ask her to put it in the shop.' He had a high frequency hearing loss. By watching gestures, lip reading and hearing the vowel sounds, he understood the first part of the message, but was completely at a loss to deliver the second part. This case illustrates the danger of considering a child with an apparently mild hearing loss as mentally retarded, and the necessity to test hearing in every child with a language delay.

REFERENCES

BALLANTYNE J C (1970) *Deafness*. Churchill, London

BLOOM F (1963) *Our Deaf Children*. Heinemann, London

DEPARTMENTS OF HEALTH AND SOCIAL SECURITY, EDUCATION AND SCIENCE (1971) *The Child who uses a Hearing Aid*. HMSO, London

DEPARTMENT OF HEALTH AND SOCIAL SECURITY (1971) *Deafness in Early Childhood*. HMSO, London

DOUEK E E, GIBSON W P R & HUMPHRIES K E (1973) The crossed acoustic response and objective tests of hearing. *Dev. Med. Childh. Neurol.* **16**, 32

EWING I R & EWING A W G (1954) *Speech and the Deaf Child*. Manchester University Press, Manchester

FISCH L (1957) The importance of auditory communication. *Arch. Dis. Childh.* **32**, 163, 230

FISCH L (1969) *Notes on High Frequency Hearing Loss in Children*. London Borough of Harringay

FRASER G R, FROGGATT P & JAMES T N (1964) Congenital deafness associated with electrocardiographic abnormalities. *Quart. J. Med.* **33**, 361

KNUDSER P (1966) *What is Special Education?* Proc. 1st Int. Conf. Ass. Spec. Educ., London

McCALL R F (1960) *Hearing Loss Hearing Aids*. South-East Association for Deaf, Bedford

REED M (1960) *Hearing Test Cards*. RNID, London

REED M (1970) Deaf and partially hearing children. In *The Psychological Assessment of Mental and Physical Handicaps*, ed. P Mittler. Methuen, London

SHERIDAN M (1968) *Stycar Hearing Test*. National Foundation for Educational Research, London

VAN DEN HOEVE (1966) *3rd International Seminar on Special Education, Germany*

WHETNALL E & FRY D B (1971) *The Deaf Child*. Heinemann, London

Chapter 4
Management of the Child with a Severe Hearing Loss

Incidence

It is estimated that 6 out of every 10,000 school children in Britain attend a special school for so-called deaf children. There are a further 2·5 per 10,000 children attending Partial Hearing Units attached to ordinary schools. This means that 8·5 per 10,000 school children are having special help with education because of defective hearing. This figure will not include the fairly high number of children who are mentally severely subnormal and attend training schools, or are resident in hospitals for the subnormal, and who also have a hearing loss. There will also be a comparable number of children under school age. This adds up to a figure of between 30,000 and 40,000 children in England and Wales who require help because of hearing loss.

MANAGEMENT

This is based on two facts. First, very few children with a hearing problem are totally deaf; and their residual hearing, however minimal, can be used to encourage understanding of language. Secondly, most children with a severe hearing loss learn to lip read. These two factors mean that many deaf children can learn to understand and to speak. This approach is called 'oralism'.

Oralism

From early babyhood a normally hearing child is learning, by his hearing, a tremendous amount about his environment. He soon learns to distinguish sounds such as his mother's voice, and the preparation of his feeds. Later on, he babbles and hears adults responding to his babble and his early intonations. This leads on to early speech patterns, and later to speech. But several months before a small child has developed speech, he has a considerable under-standing of simple language, gained from oft repeated words spoken by those around him. The deaf child is cut off from all this early experience. He lives from babyhood in a lonely, silent world. Because he cannot hear his experiences are limited to his field of vision. He does not hear his mother coming. She appears suddenly. He cannot hear her moving near him. He thinks she has gone away. He cannot understand situations that require hearing, such as his mother suddenly leaving him to answer the door. Unless the mother and the family are helped to understand what the hearing defect means to the child, and how he can be helped, he will become very emotionally disturbed, withdrawn and often aggressive. If this deprivation continues into childhood he may never develop a fully mature understanding of language. He may have no inner thought, even though he may fundamentally have a good intelligence.

For these reasons every avenue must be explored to give the child understanding and language. Even though there is no apparent response to very loud noises, it must not be presumed that he has no hearing at all. The mother should be encouraged to speak very loudly into his ears with the language she would use to a normal baby. At an early age the child should be fitted with a hearing aid, which he should wear for a short time each day. While he is wearing it, the room (preferably a carpeted one) should be quiet, and the sounds that he hears should be meaningful. The radio or television should not be a continuous background noise. At the same time the mother should let the baby see her face, so that he can also develop the ability to lip read. This training is essentially done by the mother within the family circle. She must have support to carry on this work. In many areas the family is visited frequently by a teacher for the young deaf child, who takes him for periods of auditory training and helps the mother with the training. It is hoped that in this way the child will develop some speech.

Nursery School

Ideally at the age of $2\frac{1}{2}$–3 years the child should have an opportunity to play and communicate with children of his own age. This may be in a nursery group, or it may be felt that the child needs extra help in a preschool group for the deaf.

School Placement

At the age of 5 years, or earlier, the decision must be made as to whether the child needs provision for the 'deaf' or for the 'partial hearing'. The Ministry of Education (1962) defines the two conditions:

1 *Deaf pupils* are pupils with impaired hearing who require education by methods suitable for pupils with little or no naturally acquired speech or language.

2 *Partially hearing pupils* are pupils with impaired hearing whose development of speech and language, even if retarded, is following a normal pattern, and who require for their education special arrangements or facilities, though not necessarily all the educational methods used for deaf pupils.

Children in the second category should be placed in a unit for partially hearing pupils attached to a normal school. It is hoped that with the use of a hearing aid many will be able to attend normal school.

Reed (1964) gives the four main differences in approach to the education of the deaf and partially hearing as:

		Deaf	*Partially hearing*
1	Communication	Lip reading rather than hearing	Hearing rather than lip reading
2	Rate of communication	Slower	Faster
3	Language	Artificially built up	Stimulated more incidentally
4	Speech	Largely taught artificially	Only speech defects need attention

For them, the teacher needs the following type of instructions.

1 The hard of hearing child should be seated in a front seat (with his better ear towards the teacher if there is deafness in one ear only), or in a favourable position if seats are not arranged in rows.

2 The child should be allowed to watch the face of the teacher when she is talking to the class.

3 When speaking to the class, the teacher should try to face the hard of hearing child as much as possible and to give important instructions from a position close to the child.

4　The hard of hearing child should be allowed, and encouraged, to turn round so as to see the faces of children participating in class activities. He should also be allowed to turn round when the teacher is not in front of him.

5　The teacher should avoid using loud tones or exaggerated lip movements in speaking to the child.

6　If a choice of teachers is possible, the hard of hearing child should be placed with the teacher who speaks slowly and precisely.

7　We are apt to overestimate the hearing efficiency of the child, because, when he pays attention, he apparently hears quite well. Remember that this child must use more effort to hear than the one who hears normally. It is to be expected that it will be hard to hold the attention of this child.

8　A hearing loss lasting over a period of time tends to result in a dull voice and inaccurate diction. Encourage the hard of hearing child to speak clearly.

9　Interest in music should be encouraged, especially participation in vocal music.

10　Since a hearing loss is a defect which affects the language process, the child should be encouraged to compensate by a more active interest in all language activities; reading, spelling, etc.

11　The hard of hearing child should be watched carefully to see that he is not withdrawing from the group, and that he is not suffering a personality reaction as a direct result of his impairment.

12　The hard of hearing child should be handled so as not to call attention to the defect.

13　Most hard of hearing children benefit greatly from using a hearing aid. If a child has been given an aid, he should wear it all the time during lessons. Even with a hearing aid, all the above suggestions are still very important.

Special Schools for the Hard of Hearing

Others will need more specialised help in a school for the deaf, or more correctly for the child with a severe hearing loss, where several forms of equipment will help him with his difficulty.

Hearing Aid

The hearing aid consists of three parts, the microphone, the amplifier which makes use of transistors, and the receiver. In the normal type of hearing aid issued through the National Health Service to children in Britain (the Medresco Aid), the microphone and amplifier are in a small pack which can be worn in a bag or clipped on to the child's clothing; and the receiver is fitted into the earpiece. The microphone should face outwardly and be covered by light clothing only. The receiver is attached to the amplifier by battery leads, which pass under the clothing and round to the back of the ear. The receiver is clipped into an ear mould which fits tightly into the ear. The ear mould must be made specifically for each individual child, so that there is a perfect fit. The mould is made of acrylic material after an impression of the ear, using a material such as zelgan, has been taken by an audiometrician in the local audiology clinic. The hearing aid should not be used unless the ear mould fits snugly. In some cases the rubbing of clothing distorts the hearing aid, or the aid may be damaged by an active child. In these cases a postaural aid can be supplied in which microphone, amplifier and receiver are all contained in the same insert and attached to the ear mould. In other cases, a hearing aid attached to a spectacle frame may be used. In rare instances, the ear mould may cause eczema of the external meatus; and in occasional cases there may be stenosis of the meatus. In these situations a bone-conduction receiver must be used, which is worn attached to a band over the head.

A hearing aid must have a hand-operated volume control attached so that the user can turn down the sound if near the speaker, or amplify it if listening from a distance. Aids should have a built-in automatic volume control. This is particularly needed for perceptive deafness, where a loud sound may become painful to the ear. The method used is called 'peak clipping'. This method automatically 'clips' the peak of loud intensity waves and will prevent the sounds becoming too loud, but it causes some distortion. There is no such thing as a perfect hearing aid; and some people with perceptive deafness may find them unpleasant to use.

In some cases it is recommended that a child should wear a hearing aid in both ears. If the hearing loss is different in both ears, two separate aids will be needed and may be bulky. Some workers advocate binaural aids to improve the child's hearing in an enlarged environment. Other workers think differently. First, by the use of residual hearing in the ear not wearing an aid, the child learns to cut out extraneous noises. Secondly, there is the evidence that a loud amplification of sound may actually damage the acoustic pathways, and over a period of time the child's hearing may deteriorate; for this reason it is better to have an aid in one ear only.

It must be realised that the child is given an aid not only to hear other people's voices, but also to hear himself and to get a feedback from his own voice, which will help him to correct his own speech.

Every child who is given a hearing aid needs supervision. A teacher for the deaf, or other qualified person, should be with the child for the first few sessions when the aid is worn, and should help him to listen to meaningful sounds. The aid should be worn only in a quiet room and not in the street; and people speaking to the child should be close to him. Extraneous noises in the house should at first be reduced to a minimum.

Instructions on how to care for the hearing aid must be given in writing. There are various pamphlets available. A booklet *The Child who uses a Hearing Aid* has been issued by the Departments of Health and Social Security and Education and Science. Advice on helping the child, and also on the care of batteries, the cleaning of the ear mould etc., are given.

Every child wearing a hearing aid should be seen at an audiology clinic every six months to check that the aid is working satisfactorily. The ears must be examined for wax or any infection. The child's hearing must be tested to make sure he is benefiting from the use of the aid. General encouragement must be given.

Induction Loop

This device is used in classrooms where active children are wearing hearing aids. The child's body-worn aid picks up the sounds from a loop of wire laid round the walls. The teacher speaks into a microphone to which an amplifier is attached, and the sound is picked up by the child's aid so that he can hear amplified speech in any part of the room.

Speech Trainer

This is used to train individual children, and can be used by the speech therapist or teacher. The child wears earphones. The speech sounds produced are louder and clearer than those heard with a normal hearing aid. The child can also listen to his own voice more easily by the use of an individual microphone.

Group Hearing Aid

With this apparatus, a group of older children can sit round a table, each wearing headphones, and hear sounds of greater clarity and wider frequencies. They also have individual microphones to talk to each other (figure 4.1).

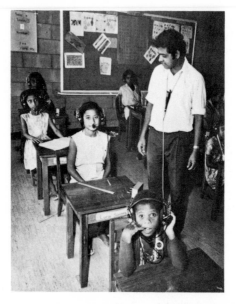

Fig. 4.1 Deaf children in a class using a group hearing aid. They are lip reading instructions from the photographer. (By kind permission of the Headmaster of Suva Crippled Children School, Fiji)

Some schools are now using a 'Radio Link' by which the child hears the teacher's voice at a considerable distance, for instance in the corridors and play ground.

Adapters to Radio and Television

Adapters can be fitted to a set so that an individual picks up the sounds in his own hearing aid at a louder amplitude, without interfering with the listening of the other members of the family.

Education

In a special school for these children an ordinary curriculum can be carried out; and many deaf children can take part in an academic education. It has been found that the child who is born deaf is at a disadvantage when compared with a child who became deaf during childhood. The born-deaf child, given much early help, may still not develop the inner language and understanding necessary to do well in an academic world, although there have been marked exceptions. This accentuates the value of very early auditory training. If a child becomes deaf at the age of 6 months, he has had, even in those early months, a head start on a born-deaf child. It is therefore imperative to give the born-deaf child very early help.

If a child becomes deaf due to meningitis, accident or some other cause, an effort must be made to retain the speech he already has and to prevent a deterioration. As soon as he is well enough after the catastrophe, he should have auditory training and a hearing aid, and should be helped to continue using his speech, or this can be lost.

THE CHILD WITH
ADDITIONAL HANDICAPS

It has been stressed that the majority of handicapped children are multiply handicapped. Possibly in the field of hearing defects we see more children with the single handicap than in the other fields of handicap. In schools for the deaf there are many children with deafness only. This appears to make it difficult to place children with hearing loss and an additional handicap in these schools. As was shown when we were discussing aetiology, deafness may be associated with cerebral palsy, blindness and mental subnormality. The child with cerebral palsy and a partial hearing loss is often an intelligent child, as this double handicap occurs more often in the athetoid form of cerebral palsy. This child needs help with the motor handicap and the hearing loss. There must be full facilities for the teaching of the partially deaf in schools for the physically handicapped, or these children must be catered for in schools for the partially hearing. This emphasises the responsibility that falls on teachers in special schools to make facilities for all types of handicaps. The blind-deaf child is a separate problem, and will be discussed in a separate chapter.

Children with a partial hearing loss may be mentally severely subnormal with an IQ under 50, or educationally subnormal. The first group includes children with Down's syndrome, gargoylism and cerebral palsy, who usually attend training schools. These children should have the regular services of a teacher of the deaf, and should gradually be helped to use a hearing aid.

The children who are partially hearing and of a level of intelligence in the range 50–70 present their own special problems. It is difficult to get an estimate of the intelligence of a young deaf child; and psychologists have to rely on performance tests. There will be children with a hearing loss due to brain pathology who also have the perceptual and learning difficulties of so-called brain-damaged children. Some of them will be hyperactive and distractible; and many will have a superadded emotional disturbance. These children will not fit into the same classes as the single-handicap deaf child. They may need a special class or a special school similar to the one run by the Royal National Institute for the Deaf, Larchmoor School in Berkshire.

MANUALISM

A problem arises when severely hearing impaired children are unable to master lip reading and the *oral* approach to education is a failure. Unless something is done to help them they will be left without a means of communication. As adults they will be solitary and unemployable, and will end up in some form of residential institution, often a hospital for the mentally subnormal.

When it has been proved that children are not learning oral methods of communication, a manual form of communication should be taught. This subject arouses a considerable amount of emotion. Deaf adults often feel very strongly that they should have been taught manual communication, so that later they can communicate with each other more readily. The argument against this is that it tends to isolate the deaf in communities of their own, leaving them out of touch with hearing people.

These arguments break down when we are dealing with children who are not learning to communicate at all. There are several 'sign' languages; and this in itself causes confusion. In fact it has been said that a trained person can tell which school for the deaf an adult attended as a child by his sign language. The Royal National Institute for the Deaf have a sign language which can be readily learnt by the deaf and by people working with them. It tends to be a concrete simplified form of language. A more grammatical sign language is in the process of being formulated by Lady Paget and Pierre Gorman, and this may form a basis for communication which it is said should lead on to a better understanding of normal grammatical language through lip reading and hearing aids.

A third very simplified form of sign language has been worked out for the severely subnormal child with cerebral palsy by Levitt (1970). This is intended to give the child a chance to express needs such as a desire for a drink, or to go to the toilet; and it should lead on to further communication.

Finger Spelling

This is a more sophisticated form of manual communication used by older children and adults to communicate with each other. It can be learnt by normal hearing people such as social workers for the deaf. It can be used in combination with a sign language; and it obviously requires a knowledge of reading.

The practice varies in different countries. In special schools for the deaf in New South Wales, Australia, finger spelling is introduced into the curriculum at eight years of age. In America a method of finger spelling using one hand only has been introduced, where the teacher speaks or writes on the board and uses finger spelling at the same time.

Educational Alternatives

The education of the child with a severe hearing loss may therefore take place in many ways: in the home with the mother helped by a preschool teacher for the deaf; in a nursery school for children with a similar handicap; in a normal school; in a school for the partially hearing; in a special class for the children with hearing loss attached to a normal school. There are also grounds for suggesting that each

Chapter 4

special school for children with a severe hearing loss should have two additional sections, one for the partially hearing educationally subnormal child, and one for the partially hearing mentally severely subnormal child.

REFERENCES

DEPARTMENT OF EDUCATION AND SCIENCE (1968) *The Education of Deaf Children.* HMSO, London

EWING I R & EWING A W G (1961) *New Opportunities for Deaf Children.* University of London Press, London

LEVITT L M A (1970) *A Method of Communication for Non-speaking Severely Subnormal Children.* Spastics Society, London

MINISTRY OF EDUCATION (1962) *Children with Impaired Hearing,* Circ. 10/62. HMSO, London

REED M (1964) Principles of education for the deaf and partially hearing. *The Child who does not Talk. Clinics in Developmental Medicine,* No. 13. Spastics Society & William Heinemann, London

REED M (1970) *Deaf and Partially Hearing Children. The Psychological Assessment of Mental and Physical Handicaps.* Methuen, London

WHETNALL E & FRY D B (1970) *Learning to Hear.* Heinemann, London

Chapter 5
The Blind Child

The title of this chapter highlights the difference between the visually handicapped and the hearing handicapped child. In discussing the child with a severe hearing loss, it is emphasised that few of these children have a total hearing loss, and management is aimed at making use of the residual hearing. Many visually handicapped children are totally blind; and they must be trained by methods that make no allowance for sight.

A separate group are children who have partial sight and can learn by visual means. They require different educational provision from the totally blind child.

However the classifications are blurred in this field as in the field of hearing. Some children who need education as blind children have some sight. Their sight may only enable them to distinguish between light and dark; but it may be of great assistance in moving around and avoiding objects. Some may have sufficient sight to distinguish large objects. This gives them a sense of size, shape, depth, distance, height, and often a dim perception of colour. With this amount of sight a child may be able to recognise visually a familiar person, such as his mother. This sensory appreciation can make a difference to his mobility, his understanding of the world and his idea of body image. It is possible that with training, and as he gets older, his use of this minimal visual ability will increase.

As will be noted when aetiology is considered, blindness may develop during childhood or adolescence, and the child may progress from a normal school through a school for the visually handicapped to a school for the blind. Some of these childhood diseases involve cerebral deterioration; and the intelligence may deteriorate.

In a high proportion of cases of blindness in children in developed countries, the condition is associated with additional handicaps, cerebral palsy, epilepsy, a hearing loss or mental subnormality.

In general, a child with visual acuity of 3/60 (Snellen) or less is considered blind, and in Britain is registered as such from early childhood.

DETECTION OF VISUAL LOSS

This will be detected at birth if there is a gross abnormality of the eyes, such as anophthalmos, microphthalmos or bilateral cataracts. In the neonatal period, vision can be tested in a few simple ways. If the pupils do not react to light, there are grounds for concern; but an intact pupillary reflex only shows that the eye and optic pathways to the lateral geniculate body are intact. It does not test cortical vision. A new-born baby will blink if a light is shone in the eye. André Thomas (1960) has shown that an alert baby of one week old will open his eyes if slowly turned away from a source of light and will turn his head to keep facing it. From the early weeks, the normal baby will focus on an object. The incoordinated eye movements noted soon after birth disappear, the eyes move synchronously and purposefully, and the child looks at his mother and interesting, meaningful objects.

It is when these signs of normal development are not taking place that the parents begin to worry. If there is a visual handicap, the delay in this field will be pinpointed by comparing the baby's development with the normal on developmental tests.

If there is any concern the child should be referred to an ophthalmologist. If a total loss of vision is suspected the child can be tested by *visual evoked response*. The electroencephalogram is recorded before and during the time that the child receives a light stimulus from a stroboscope. No alteration in rhythm and a flat curve indicate a total loss of sight.

If a deterioration of sight occurs during childhood, it may be noted by parents or teacher, or reported by the child himself. Lack of progress at school, or a change in behaviour, may be the first signs.

The development of a squint, or a wandering eye which fails to focus, may be the first indication that sight has been lost in that eye. This may be the earliest sign of a condition such as retinoblastoma.

All children with a visual handicap should also see a paediatrician, and usually a paediatric neurologist, as often other systems are involved. The paediatrician should be involved in advice and management and ongoing support of the family.

AETIOLOGY

Blindness in children may be caused by maldevelopment or damage to different parts of the eye, the optic nerves or the visual nerve pathways to the occipital lobe. Possibly in as many as 50% of cases at present in developed countries, the condition is genetic in origin, either autosomal dominant, sex-linked dominant or autosomal recessive. Abnormal genetic endowment may account for abnormalities in any part of the visual apparatus, cornea, lens, iris, retina, choroid or optic nerve pathways. As many as 19 autosomal dominant, 30 autosomal recessive and 10 sex-linked genetic entities are known as the causation of childhood blindness.

Other causes are maternal infection or drugs in early pregnancy, prematurity, perinatal illness, postnatal ocular and cerebral infections, eye tumours and injuries, detachment of the retina, cerebral tumour and deteriorating neurological conditions.

The commonest groups of conditions are discussed briefly.

Congenital Abnormalities

Anophthalmos, Microphthalmos and Coloboma

The child may be born with obvious congenital abnormalities of the eyes, and immediately it can be seen that he has useless vestigial remnants of the eyes. Or he may show aniridia—absent irides— colobomata of the iris or retina, or fibrotic vestigial remains in the eye. The condition may be associated with cataracts.

The child with the condition may be the only affected member of the family. There is a possibility of dominant inheritance with variable clinical expression in some cases. Sjögren and Larsson (1949) reported a large series in Sweden. There may have been very early damage to the developing fetus. Drugs in pregnancy, such as antithyroid drugs and thalidomide, have been the cause. In 50% of cases the child also shows mental retardation.

Toxoplasmosis in the mother can cause abnormalities of this type. Apart from microphthalmos there is often hydrocephalus or microcephalus, and X-ray evidence of intracerebral calcification. The serum of any baby with microphthalmos should be tested serologically for toxoplasmosis. A titre above 1 : 16 under 11 years is very significant. A condition of choroidoretinitis, due to maternal infection, may begin in infancy and is amenable to treatment.

Cataracts

Congenital opacities of the lens occur in children in a wide variety of clinical conditions. The single abnormality of congenital cataract may be genetically dominant or recessive. It occurs also in genetically and biochemically determined conditions such as galactosaemia (the cataract may be present at birth or develop in later life); the syndrome of Lowe, Terrey and MacLachlan, which includes a renal tubal defect, vitamin resistant rickets and mental subnormality; and Hallerman-Strieff syndrome, where there is a birdlike face, dwarfism, blue sclerae and deficiency of hair growth. Cataracts occur quite commonly in Down's syndrome, sometimes developing in childhood and adolescence. Rare conditions are Werner's syndrome, where there is a diffuse scleroderma; and Marinesco-Sjögren syndrome, in which there is, in addition, spinocerebellar atrophy. Cataracts are seen quite frequently in patients in hospitals for the mentally subnormal, and may be associated with abnormally shaped skulls. Cataracts may develop during childhood or adolescence in conditions such as dystrophia myotonica.

Non-genetic forms of cataracts may follow maternal toxaemia and occur in babies of low birthweight. It was shown by McDonald (1964) that these children may be light for dates rather than premature by dates. Hypoglycaemia may cause the lens damage. This group of children often have additional handicaps such as cerebral palsy, epilepsy and mental retardation.

Rubella

Perhaps the commonest cause of congenital cataract today is rubella infection in the mother in the first two months of pregnancy. All infants with cataracts should be tested for rubella antibodies. At birth, the antibody titre for mother and baby will be the same. If there has been a rubella infection of the baby in fetal life the titre will remain at the same level, or will show a rise at a few months of age. If there has been no rubella infection, the titre will fall rapidly. These cases tend to be born in the autumn, after a spring infection in the mother. The eyes are often small, and there may be an associated retinitis. The children also show other abnormalities. Deafness may occur if the infection was somewhat later in pregnancy. Microcephaly, congenital heart defect, cerebral palsy of a rigid type and epilepsy may be associated. There is often superadded mental deficiency. Many of these children are restless, hyperactive and extraordinarily agile. Many appear to be as happy standing on their heads as the right way up. Objective tests of hearing may show that they can hear, but suffer from a lack of auditory discrimination. Neither everyday sounds nor words have any meaning for them. Their inability to make contact with other children or with adults leads to severe behaviour disorders, tantrums, screaming attacks, damaging property, such as breaking windows, and other forms of aggressiveness. Some people might describe them as autistic.

Some children are less severely involved, and can be trained as suggested in the chapter on the deaf-blind child.

Treatment for Cataracts

This condition may be compared with conductive deafness. If the retina and optic nerve pathways are intact, it is important to give the child the opportunity to use his sight as soon as possible, or the eyes will become amblyopic. If the cataracts are bilateral and total or very extensive, early surgery should be considered. If the cataracts are partial, it may be wiser to postpone surgery, as the operation is not as successful with children as with adults. In cases of rubella, the virus may still be dormant in the lens. An infection may develop after surgery, leading to total loss of vision due to enophthalmitis. It may be preferable to operate on one eye in early life and on the other later.

After surgery for cataracts the child is hypermetropic and unable to accommodate. Glasses of 10–14 dioptres must be worn constantly. Contact lenses can be worn by children. In cases of partial cataract, an enlarged field of vision may be obtained by frequent use of homatropine drops or by iridectomy.

Optic Atrophy

There are three distinct forms of optic atrophy which may cause a severe visual handicap in childhood.

There may be a congenital abnormality of the optic disc, with hypoplasia of the optic nerve. The disc is misshapen, small and white. The condition is a recessive or very occasionally a dominant condition, and various forms have been described. The syndrome has been called Leber's optic atrophy.

Secondly, optic atrophy may be found in children following a cerebral insult, either perinatal damage or a later infective illness. After a premature birth or a stormy neonatal period, the child has a delay in acquiring the ability to focus his eyes and has incoordinated eye movements. On examination the optic discs show marked pallor. Other evidence of neurological damage, such as cerebral palsy, epilepsy and/or mental retardation, is noted. In some of these children, as they grow older, it may become apparent that there is a considerable amount of sight. A child reported as blind at birth may crawl to pick up a sweet, and will come into the category of the partially sighted. The same sequence of events may follow a cerebral infection, when it has been thought that there has been a total loss of vision.

Thirdly, optic atrophy may develop in deteriorating neurological syndromes such as the leucodystrophies, cerebral lipidoses and hereditary ataxias. It may also develop in children with hydrocephalus and other types of abnormally shaped skulls, and in craniostenosis.

Cerebral Blindness

Some brain-damaged children may behave as though they have no vision, and yet the eyes and the optic discs are normal. In these cases, the blindness may be due to damage to the occipital cortex, and the blindness is *cerebral* in origin. Often the occiput is flat and there are other signs of severe cerebral involvement. Total blindness can be confirmed by retinal evoked response electroencephalography.

Buphthalmos

This condition is due to a congenital abnormality of the filtration angle of the anterior chamber. The condition as a separate entity is inherited as an autosomal recessive and several siblings may be affected. The cornea becomes blurred from corneal oedema due to increased pressure in the eye. The cornea increases in diameter and the child shows signs of photophobia. Sight may be preserved by surgical treatment—a goniotomy operation. An incision is made into the anterior chamber and a sweep with a knife is made through the fibrous tissue to open up the angle.

Glaucoma

This condition may develop in the neonatal period, or later, in children with dislocated lens or aniridia.

Tumours

Retrolental Fibroplasia

This condition was first described by Terry (1942); many cases occurred up to 1955, and unfortunately quite a number since that date. All the children involved were premature by weight and by dates—many under three pounds at birth. They had been exposed to a level of oxygen of 60–70% in an incubator, and then suddenly released into a normal oxygen-containing environment. The condition is caused by a proliferation of retinal vessels, which become fibrosed, cause retinal detachment and fill the inner chamber of the eye with a fibrous mass. In most cases the condition is bilateral, and leads to total blindness. Some residual vision may be preserved.

Pseudoglioma (Norrie's disease)

This is a non-malignant disturbance caused by a detachment of the retina in the perinatal or early postnatal period. An ill-defined fibrous mass develops in the inner chamber. There is evidence of a sex-linked recessive inheritance.

Retinoblastoma

This is the commonest malignant tumour affecting the eyes in childhood. It is noticed in the first 6 years of life, usually before 2 years of age. The tumours arise from the retina. The first sign may be a squint, particularly a deviating eye. If the tumour is detected early, radiation can arrest its development. In many cases the eye must be enucleated. The second eye may be involved not by an extension of the tumour, but by the development of a new tumour. Total blindness in a once-seeing child results. If left, the condition is fatal. Some cases arise sporadically, but in about 40% of them the mother or father has had the condition. It is inherited as a pure dominant and the chance of an affected adult having an affected child is 1:2. Children of affected parents should be seen by an ophthalmologist at very frequent intervals. Many of these children have an above-average intelligence.

Retinal Aplasia
(Leber's tapeto-retinal dystrophies)

Leber originally described these conditions in 1916; and under this heading are included a wide range of diseases which involve a disturbance of pigmentation of the retina with choroidoretinal degeneration.

Retinal aplasia may cause blindness or defective sight from birth or it may develop in childhood without evidence of any other handicapping condition. Pigmentary changes in the retina are noted when the evidence of defective sight is established, but could have been detected earlier by a diminished response to electroretinography (Harcourt 1971). The pigmentation may later involve the macula, and optic atrophy, narrowing of retinal vessels and choroidal sclerosis may occur.

The early signs in the later form are night blindness, and later peripheral and central field defects. The condition is inherited as an autosomal recessive and consanguinity in the parents has been reported.

Pigmentary retinal changes may also occur in association with other handicapping conditions. Children with the combined handicaps of blindness and mental retardation were described by Sorsby & Williams (1960). In Batten-Mayou disease, a normal child may show deteriorating sight, followed by intellectual deterioration leading to total idiocy. Syndromes such as Laurence-Moon-Bardet-Biedl and Friedreich's ataxia may also show retinitis. A benign form which does not usually cause total blindness in childhood is retinitis pigmentosa (Usher's syndrome) associated with a hearing loss. Albinism might also come under this heading.

The occurrence of this disease in association with other handicaps emphasises the importance of an ophthalmological examination for all handicapped children. In one assessment centre four cases of this type were found in six months.

Other Causes of Childhood Blindness

Blindness may occur due to corneal clouding in some forms of gargoylism, or as a result of a dislocated lens in Marfan's syndrome or homocystinuria.

Maternal syphilis is a rare cause of blindness today but is suspected in any case of juvenile interstitial keratitis.

Children with Still's disease may develop iridocyclitis. They may go blind due to glaucoma or cataract.

Intracranial tumour can cause loss of sight. Craniopharyngioma is the commonest brain tumour resulting in blindness in childhood. The tumour causes a bitemporal hemianopia, and symptoms of raised intracranial pressure. The child complains of headache and poor vision. If the tumour is diagnosed early, the sight may improve due to release of the pressure on the optic chiasma.

Accidents such as firework injuries are the cause of some cases of blindness in special schools for the blind.

Ophthalmia neonatorum is a rare cause of blindness in Britain today; but it is still common in developing countries. Possibly in nine-tenths of the world the commonest cause of blindness is trachoma. In both cases the blindness is due to corneal scarring.

ADDITIONAL HANDICAPS

It is generally agreed that the majority of blind children in Britain today have additional handicaps.

Mental Retardation

A lowered intelligence may occur in many types of visual defect, but it is particularly liable to be present when the visual handicap is due to antenatal and perinatal abnormalities, or postnatal involvement of the cerebral cortex in injury or infection. In contrast, it has been found that in retinoblastoma, buphthalmos and some forms of

Chapter 5

retinal dysplasia, the intelligence may be above average. There are often exceptions to this finding, and the author has met two children with retinoblastoma and mental subnormality.

The difference in the aetiology of blindness in children attending schools for the blind and in a group of children with the double handicap of severe visual defects and mental subnormality (IQ below 50) is illustrated by table 5.1.

In the mentally subnormal group there is a higher incidence of cases due to prenatal infection, optic atrophy and microphthalmos. In the educable group there is an increase in cases due to retinoblastoma, myopia, aniridia and choroidoretinal degeneration. The cases acquired in infancy are of an entirely different aetiology in the two groups. The 12 children with acquired blindness in the Woods group all had optic atrophy following meningitis or other cerebral causes. The cases in the educable group were due to accidents, inflammation, tumours and vascular conditions. Of the 126 mentally subnormal children, 60 were premature by weight.

Table 5.1   Difference in the Aetiology of Blindness in Mentally Subnormal Children and Children Attending Special Schools

Type	Woods Survey (mentally subnormal children)		Fraser Survey (children attending special schools)	
	No.	%	No.	%
Retrolental fibroplasia	20	16·6	177	22·9
Optic atrophy (perinatal)	18	14·1	56	7·2
Cataract	22	17·5	107	13·8
Retinoblastoma	0	0	43	5·6
Pseudoglioma	4	3·3	25	3·2
Myopia—retinal detachment	1	0·9	22	2·9
Microphthalmos anophthalmos	9	7·8	25	3·2
Buphthalmos	4	3·3	39	5·0
Antenatal infection	16	10·1	17	2·3
Aniridia	0	0	11	1·5
Lesions of cornea	0	0	6	0·8
Choroidoretinal degeneration	8	6·5	116	14·9
Degenerating conditions	4	3·2	0	0
Associated malformations	8	6·5	55	7·0
Acquired in infancy (meningitis, hydrocephalus, battered babies)	12	10·4	77	9·9
	126	100·0	776	100·0

Cerebral Palsy

Cerebral palsy of all forms may accompany severe visual loss. Optic atrophy and blindness may occur where there has been damage to both parieto-occipital pathways, as in bilateral hemiplegia. With this double handicap, mental retardation is almost an inevitable third handicap, but cases of normal intelligence are known. Cataracts may be an additional handicap, where cerebral palsy is associated with a premature birth or maternal toxaemia. Retrolental fibroplasia and spastic diplegia (Little's disease), both caused by a severely premature birth, do not usually occur in the same child. Possibly oxygen therapy caused retrolental fibroplasia but prevented spastic diplegia.

Epilepsy may be an additional handicap in any condition which has a cerebral origin.

Partial Deafness

A severe hearing loss can occur in the rubella syndrome, following cases of prematurity and in retinitis pigmentosa. A hearing loss of even a minor degree is a serious handicap to a blind child, who must rely on his hearing to learn about his world. Blind children are liable to get upper respiratory infections as they are less mobile, and glue ears due to an unresolved otitis media readily occur. All infections must be energetically treated. Even a 20 decibel loss in hearing can cause a blind child to become very disturbed. Hearing aids should be readily available to blind children, and help if necessary from a teacher of the deaf.

Learning Problems

Brain-damaged blind children may have all the difficulties described in chapter 8. There may be body image difficulties, and a fundamental inability to understand spatial relationships. This may be a factor in a child being late in walking. Even if the hearing is good, there may be a specific defect in auditory discrimination. This may occur in children with the rubella syndrome. There may be specific language difficulties amounting to a dysphasia. However it is generally found that blind children are very verbal children. They may chatter endlessly without any specific meaning to their speech. The actual enunciation of the words may be clear; but their knowledge of language has run ahead of their experience of everyday life.

With the help of a psychologist conversant with blind children, some of these learning problems can be sorted out. For example, a right-handed child became blind and developed a right hemiplegia at the age of 4 years. He became a verbal child and gave evidence of a good intelligence. His refusal to take part in any manual occupation at school was due to the spasticity and astereognosis in his right hand. He needed specific help to learn to use his left hand, and the hemiplegia was really the major handicap.

Behaviour Disorders

Blind children tend to be inactive children who develop fluent speech and attempt to dominate their environment with continuous chatter. They may ask the same question frequently, and often their speech is echolalic. This repetitive speech militates against intellectual development, and is serious evidence of maladjustment and inappropriate early handling.

Other blind children may become withdrawn. They may retire into a corner, banging their heads on the ground and making no contact with others. When a child is behaving like this it is impossible to judge the true intelligence. Other blind children take refuge in a world of fantasy, which adults may unwittingly augment by playing with the child and his fantasy. It may be hard to break the pattern.

Some blind children can show severe temper tantrums, and become so aggressive that it is difficult to handle them. Others may show the hyperactivity and lack of concentration of the seeing brain-damaged child.

Mannerisms or Blindisms

These may occur in both intelligent and dull blind children. They take the form of incessant rocking, gyrating, eye-poking or banging the head (figure 5.1). These mannerisms are socially unacceptable and may be due partly to the fact that the child cannot see the disapproval of others. They are also evidence of his underlying frustration and of the lack of early stimulation and interest when these mannerisms first developed.

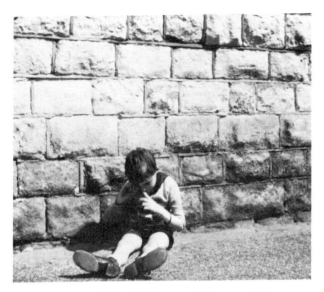

Fig. 5.1 A blind withdrawn child, head rocking.

Incidence

Fine (1968) enumerated the incidence of additional handicaps in 817 blind children who attended special schools for the blind (table 5.2). These figures did not include blind children with IQ estimated as under 50. The figures would be higher in the blind mentally subnormal.

Table 5.2 Incidence of Additional Handicaps in 817 Blind Children
(Fine 1968)

Handicap	%
Low intelligence	20
Physical disability	21
Hearing loss	9
Maladjustment	9
Speech and language difficulty	9
Epilepsy	8
Other handicaps	9
(obesity, eczema, asthma)	
Mannerisms	45

MANAGEMENT

In most cases the child has had expert ophthalmological investigation, and treatment from the first diagnosis of a visual defect. Many children have had repeated periods in hospital and possibly many operations, as in needling for cataracts. It is not uncommon to find that this is all the help the parents have received and that no support or advice has been given. The parents need help in coming to terms with the child's handicap from the beginning. Early official registration of blindness may help to set in motion channels of help for the mother.

If the child is born blind, the parents, particularly the mother, may be so shocked and depressed that the child will be given routine care only, and no attempt at stimulation will be made. This negative attitude is enhanced by the fact that the child does not look round for his mother, smile or show pleasure when she comes into the room. In fact, he may 'still' or become unduly quiet when he hears her which may be considered lack of interest.

This inactive sterile situation can go on for several years. A blind child may be found who is still bottle-fed and lying in his pram, but at the same time is able to repeat little catch phrases that have been said to him. He may give the impression of being mentally retarded although the acquisition of some speech gives a clue that he may have normal intelligence. A child with this type of early start in life has been permanently handicapped in his intellectual and emotional development. This situation is by no means uncommon in England today.

From the first diagnosis the child must either be seen regularly in his own home by a social worker knowledgeable in the training of the blind, or attend regularly with his mother at a clinic where help is given.

The mother must be helped to realise that the child may be capable of developing like normal-sighted children in all his early skills, and that he is much more like than unlike a normal child.

In the early months, the mother should be encouraged to make her presence known by simple speech; to put toys in the child's hands; to sit him up. He should learn to play with his hands and fingers, and then his toes, like a normal child of a few months. It has been suggested that bells should be put on his toes so that he gets a sense of body image. He should be put on the floor to play, and helped to pull himself up in a playpen. Blind children do not usually crawl but with help they can walk at the normal time. If a blind child does not sit up or walk at the normal time, he will be using his hands to balance himself when he should be using them for play.

Feeding should be as normal as possible. Weaning and change to solid food should occur at 4–8 months, and at 6 months a rusk should be put in his hand to encourage him to feed himself. Later on he should be encouraged to use a spoon, however messily. It has been suggested that blind children should be fed by someone from behind, so that they sense where the spoon comes from and are encouraged to take it themselves. In the same way with walking, an adult may help the child by holding him from behind, so that he develops the courage to go forth into the unknown. Toilet training and learning to dress and undress should take place in a normal way. A blind child will usually pick up speech quickly. It is important that he uses meaningful speech, and does not endlessly

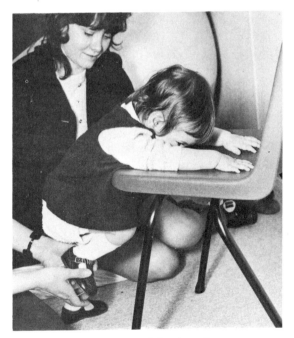

Fig. 5.2 A blind child. The mother is being shown how to encourage normal movement by a physiotherapist.

repeat nursery rhymes or what he hears on television. Part of his play should take place in a very quiet room so that he learns to rely on his hearing.

During these early years, the mother must have support to carry on and use her own ideas. Sometimes a visit for actual therapy may help a worried mother. A physiotherapist may help a child with walking, and an occupational therapist may help with encouraging everyday living activities, and give advice about training and about playthings in the home (figures 5.2 and 5.3).

Play is one of the most important factors in any young child's life, and particularly in that of a blind child. Advice about playthings is given in booklets published by the Royal National Institute for the Blind. The playthings should have real meaning. It is better to have a real cup than a doll's cup. The mother must let the child take part

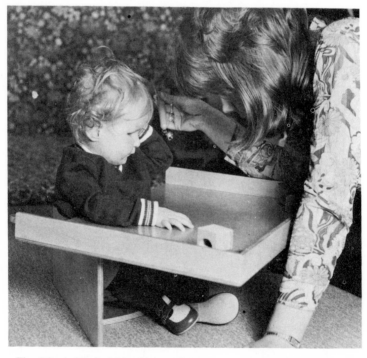

Fig. 5.3 A blind child with anophthalmos is learning to make sound discriminations with a speech therapist. She is sitting in a triangular floor seat with a tray.

in the life of the home, washing up and going to the shops. He should be encouraged to experiment with sand, water and other materials. Above everything else, he must have ample opportunities to explore. His sense of touch can be developed by playthings of different textures (figure 5.4). A situation where all the toys are made of plastic should be avoided.

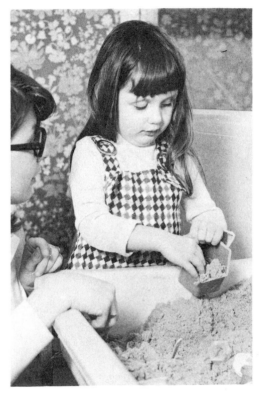

Fig. 5.4 A blind child is being shown how to enjoy normal play by an occupational therapist.

During this early period the mother should not leave the child for long periods and arrangements in the past by which the blind child left home early for special training, are now frowned upon. But at $2\frac{1}{2}$–3 years he may benefit from attendance at a normal nursery school, where he can learn social behaviour with sighted children. Excessive noise may at first be frightening him.

EDUCATION AT SCHOOL

Most blind children attend schools for the blind at the age of 5 years or earlier. As blindness is a rare handicap, many children will live at a distance from the school and will have to be resident. Every effort should be made to see that they go home every weekend.

Schools for the blind attempt a normal education. However, to learn the Braille form of reading, an IQ of about 80 is needed, so that a number of retarded blind children do not learn in this way. Blind children can be helped with individual tape recorders which record lessons, and also can use them to record their answers. In this way a teaching machine can be used for the blind. Blind children should be in close contact with children at schools for the sighted, and should join them for lessons, dances and socials. Some children may be transferred to schools for the sighted. All activities such as cooking, woodwork, keeping pets and swimming should be part of the curriculum. Every effort should be made to encourage independence, going about alone on buses and to the shops.

Children who are below average intelligence can take part in most of this activity.

In handling blind children, the staff should be continually on the alert to ensure that they are not missing out on everyday experience. I asked a boy of nine years, who was considered mentally subnormal, how far away he lived. He said, 'It's yards . . . it's minutes . . . it's miles.' He had obviously got an idea of distance, but had never been helped to understand it and its measurements. Another boy said to me 'What's soap powder? What's bleach? What's Ajax? What's soap flakes?' He had obviously made an inventory of cleaning materials from his own experience and wanted their use explained. This compiling of lists is a feature of unstimulated blind children.

At an older age the child will learn to use the long stick and the sonic torch, and be prepared for employment in the community.

THE MENTALLY RETARDED
BLIND CHILD

Undoubtedly some blind children today are mentally retarded. If there are additional handicaps, such as severe cerebral palsy and epilepsy, the retardation will be profound. In these cases the parents must be helped to give what stimulation they can to the child. They may need help with short hostel stays and baby-sitting to give them some relief. It has been felt that many blind children would not be so mentally retarded if early stimulation had been given (Woods 1968). Williams (1966) has described a blind child who was unable to walk or talk and who was incontinent at 5 years, but who later grew up to be a normal employable blind adult.

Intelligence testing in the young blind child is difficult. Several tests have been devised—the Williams adaptation of the Terman-Merrill test and the Mansfield-Buccholz Social Maturity Scale for Preschool Blind Children have been used. Possibly the best assessment is a longterm one, and the level of the child's highest attainment should be taken as his real intelligence level. While this assessment is taking place, the child should have the benefit of training in an optimum environment.

GLOSSARY OF
OPHTHALMIC TERMS

Amblyopia	Subnormal vision in a normal eye
Ametropia	Refractive error
Aniridia	Absent iris
Anisocoria	Difference in size of two pupils
Anisometropia	Difference in refractive error in two eyes
Anophthalmos	Absence of eye
Aphakia	Absence of lens
Coloboma	Notch-like defect in any of the structures of the eye or eyelid
Cycloplegia	Paralysis of the ciliary muscle resulting in loss of accommodation
Ectropion	Eversion of the eyelid
Emmetropia	No refractive error
Entropion	Inversion of the eyelid
Epiphora	Persistent overflow of tears
Esophoria	Latent tendency of eye to deviate inward
Esotropia	Inward deviation of eye
Exophoria	Latent tendency to deviate outward
Exotropia	External deviation of eye
Hypermetropia	Long sight
Hyphaema	Blood in the anterior chamber
Hypopyon	Pus in the anterior chamber
Keratoconus	Corneal atrophy giving cone-like deformity

Myopia   Short sight
Polycoria   More than one opening in the iris
Scotoma   Blind spot in a visual field
Trichiasis   Inversion of the eye lashes

REFERENCES

ANDRÉ-THOMAS A (1960) *The Neurological Examination of the Infant*. Spastics Society & William Heinemann, London

DUDGEON J A (1965) More light on rubella and congenital defects. *Dev. Med. Childh. Neurol.* 7, 196–204

ELONEN A S (1964) Appraisal of developmental lag in certain blind children. *J. Pediat.* **65**, 4, 599–610

ELONEN A S, POLZEN M & ZWARENSTEYN S B (1967) The uncommitted blind child formerly committed to institutions for the retarded. *Exceptional Children*, 306

FINE S (1968) *Blind and Partially Sighted Children*. Department of Education and Science. HMSO, London

FRASER G R & FRIEDMANN A I (1967) *The Causes of Blindness in Childhood*. Johns Hopkins Press, Baltimore

GANSTORP I (1969) *Paediatric Neurology*. Meredith, New York

GIBBS N (1966) Blind Children. *Proc. 1st Int. Conf. Ass. Spec. Educ.*, London

HARCOURT B (1971) Electroretinography as the diagnosis of tapetio-retinal degeneration. *Dev. Med. Childh. Neurol.* **12**, 775–780

LIEBMAN S D & GELLIS S (1966) *The Paediatricians' Ophthalmology*. C V & Mosby, St Louis

LOWE C V, TERREY M & MACLACHLAN E A (1952) Organic aciduria, decreased renal ammonia production, hydrophthalmos and mental retardation. *Amer. J. Dis. Child.* **83**, 164

MCDONALD A (1964) Cataract in children of a very low birth weight. *Guy's Hosp. Rep.* **1**, 113, 296

MCDONALD A (1966) Congenital cataract. *Dev. Med. Childh. Neurol.* **8**, 3.301

MANSON M, LOGAN W P D & LOYE R M (1960) *Rubella and Other Virus Infections during Pregnancy*. Ministry of Health Report No. 101 HMSO, London

NORRIE G (1927) Causes of blindness in children. *Acta ophthal.* (*Kbn.*) **5**, 357

NORRIS M, SPAULDING P J & BRODIE F H (1957) *Blindness in Childhood*. University of Chicago Press, Chicago

ROYAL NATIONAL INSTITUTE FOR THE BLIND (1966) *Training the Young Blind Child*. Information leaflet No. 9

SANDLER A M (1963) Aspects of passivity and ego development in the blind infant. The psychoanalytic study of the child. **18**, 343

SCHEIE H G, SCHAFFER D B, PLOTKIN S A & KEITESZE E D (1967) Congenital rubella cataract. *Arch. Ophthal.* **77**, 440

SELLARS S L (1969) The glue ear and rubella risk child. *Proc. roy. Soc. Med.* **62**, 2, 111

SHERIDAN M D (1964) Final report of a prospective study of children whose mothers had rubella in early pregnancy. *Brit. med. J.* **2**, 536

SJÖGREN T & LARSSON T (1949) Microphthalmos and anophthalmos with or without coincident oligophrenia. *Acta psychiat. scand*, Suppl. 56

SORSBY A & WILLIAMS C (1960) Retinal aplasia. *Brit. med. J.* **1**, 293

SORSBY A (1963) *Modern Ophthalmology.* Butterworth, London

TERRY T L (1942) Extreme prematurity and fibroblastic overgrowth of persistent vascular sheath behind each crystalline lens. *Amer. J. Ophthal.* **25**, 203

The Education of the Visually Handicapped (1972) HMSO, London

TOOMER J & COLBORN BROWN M (1963) *Blind Children Learn Through Play.* RNIB, London

WILLIAMS C (1966) A blind idiot who became a normal blind adolescent. *Dev. Med. Childh. Neurol.* **8**, 2, 166

WILLIAMS C (1968) *Psychiatric Implications of Severe Visual Defect for the Child and for the Parents. Clinics in Developmental Medicine* **32**, 110

WOODS G E (1970) The blind mentally retarded child. *Proceedings of the 2nd Congress of the International Association for the Scientific Study of Mental Deficiency, Warsaw*

Chapter 6
The Partially Sighted Child

When one sees a class of partially sighted children, and realises the difficulties they are encountering in mastering the early educational skills, and more fundamentally the difficulties they have in finding their way around, one wonders how early the disability was discovered. As physically some of these children look very normal, one suspects that in some cases the disability was not noted until late in infancy or early school life. If there is, in addition, a physical handicap such as deafness, cerebral palsy or mental subnormality, the danger of a visual handicap being missed is even greater.

For this reason, Sheridan (1969) stresses the need to test the visual acuity of all children in early life.

Vernon Smith (1969) and a team of orthoptists in Birmingham carried out a visual screening programme on 7014 children under 4 years of age, and many under 2 years. The eye defects found are given in table 6.1.

Table 6.1   Eye Defects in 7014 Children under 4 Years of Age (Vernon Smith 1969)

Defect	No.
Abnormal head posture	1
Amblyopia	11
Anisometropia	1
Buphthalmos	1
Cataract	5
Dilated pupil	1
Epiphora	41
Irregular pupil	2
Myopia	1
Nystagmus	15
Ocular palsy	11
Photophobia	8
Ptosis	21
Squint	306

TESTING OF VISION

The child's vision should be tested by the methods described in chapter 2.

Sheridan (1969) in the HMSO Pamphlet No. 102 has shown the ages at which the vision of normal children can be tested (table 6.2).

Table 6.2   Criteria for Normal vision in Children Under 5 Years
(Sheridan 1969)

Age of child	Ability
6 months	Watches 2 inch, 1 inch and $\frac{1}{2}$ inch balls at 10 feet
9 months	Watches 2 inch to $\frac{1}{4}$ inch balls at 10 feet
15 months	Watches 2 inch to $\frac{1}{8}$ inch balls at 10 feet
$2\frac{1}{2}$ years	May match VOTH at 10 feet
3 years	Recognises miniature toys at 10 feet and can do 5 letter vision test THOUX
4 years	Can recognise letters to near bottom of chart Snellen 6/9
5 years	Recognises letters at 20 feet to near bottom of chart

Other charts, used for children who are not yet able to name letters, show an E placed several ways round:

⊓ Ǝ ⊔ E

or a picture of a hand lying in the same four positions. The child must show with his own hand which way round the sign is placed. Some children may get confused with these tests.

Snellen Test

After the age of 6 years the Snellen test chart of letters of calibrated size can be used. The child's visual acuity is recorded as a fraction. Visual acuity is usually defined in terms of minimal separation, i.e. the shortest distance by which two lines can be separated and still be perceived as two lines.

Snellen letter charts are viewed at a distance of 6 metres (20 feet). The individual being tested reads aloud the smallest line he can distinguish. The results are expressed as a fraction. The numerator of the fraction is 6 (20), the distance at which the subject reads the chart. The denominator is the greatest distance from the chart at which a normal individual can read the smallest line the subject can read. Normal visual acuity is 6/6 (20/20). The Snellen charts are designed so that the height of the letters in the smallest line a normal individual can read at 6 metres (20 feet) subtends a visual angle of five minutes. Each line in the letters subtends one minute of arc and the lines in the letters are separated by one minute of arc. Thus the minimum separable in a normal individual corresponds to a visual angle of one minute. A child who can only read the top line of Snellen's chart has a vision of 6/60; and the bottom rows 6/6, 6/5 or 6/4. If the child's vision is severely affected, the largest letters may only be seen at three metres; and the vision is then 3/60. This is the worst vision at which the child is considered partially sighted. Below this level he is considered blind.

Refractive Errors

A child with mental retardation or with a severe visual loss may not have the required skill to distinguish the shapes of letters until later in childhood. If there is the slightest suspicion of a visual handicap, he should be referred to an ophthalmologist for a full examination and refraction under a mydriatic. Mongols and other mentally retarded children may not cooperate with the 5 letter test until 6 years old or later. If there is myopia this is too late to find out. There is also the danger of missing marked hypermetropia of 5 dioptres or more. These children may respond to visual testing at a distance, but near vision is not sufficient for them to learn to read. Of 20 cases of hypermetropia in one survey, there was a family history of hypermetropia in 10 cases, but no cause could be found for the rest.

AT RISK REGISTER FOR VISUAL HANDICAPS

Young children start to learn reading by using books with large letters. They appear to use a larger area of the retina. As they grow older, they use progressively smaller print and it is only at this stage that a visual handicap which has been missed may first be noticed.

Possibly there should be an 'at risk' index for children with a visual handicap and special care should be taken in the early testing of their vision. Referral to an ophthalmologist can be made as soon as difficulties are noticed. The list would include:

Children who have a parent with myopia or congenital hypermetropia

Clumsy and accident-prone children

Children with abnormal head posture

Children with a squint, nystagmus or abnormal eye movements

Children who were born prematurely

Children with a history or neurological evidence of brain pathology

Children with conditions such as Down's syndrome or muscular dystrophy (who may show myopia)

Children with specific conditions such as homocystinuria or Marfan's disease.

Definition

There is no clearcut legal or clinical definition of visual handicap, partial sightedness or subnormal vision, whichever term is used. There are certain factors which cover this group of children:

The child is using visual clues in everyday life.

The child, his parents and his teacher consider him a sighted child.

Visual acuity for distance vision may vary, but cannot be corrected to 6/12 with glasses.

Visual acuity with glasses is better than 3/60, which is the legal limit of blindness.

Central acuity may be reduced or the field of vision impaired in the presence of some normal peripheral vision.

These children can be trained to use their vision and can be educated by visual means.

AETIOLOGY

Fine (1968) analysed the causes of visual handicap in a survey of 137 children born in the years 1956–60, who attended schools for the partially sighted (table 6.3). This table does not include children with severe mental subnormality.

Table 6.3 Causes of Visual Handicap in 137 Children Born during 1956–60
(Fine 1968)

Cause	%
Cataract and lens displacement	33·27
Myopia	9·0
Optic atrophy	11·1
Nystagmus	14·0
Albinism	11·6
Disease of retina and choroid	3·7
Retrolental fibroplasia	4·1
Coloboma and developmental defects	5·8
Buphthalmos'glaucoma	2·7
Hypermetropia	1·2
Corneal lesions	2·0
Uveitis, iridocyclitis	
(due to rheumatoid arthritis)	0·7
Tumour of the eye	0·2
Cerebral blindness	0·7
	100·00

In her analysis of the causes she states that heredity accounted for 34·47%, prematurity for 10·8% and maternal infection 4·1%. In 45·6% the aetiology of the visual handicap was unknown.

The conditions that may cause partial sight are similar to those causing blindness, and all except the following four have already been discussed.

Myopia may be a familial condition, in which case the family are already alerted to watch for the defect. It is liable to occur in association with prematurity and in conditions such as Down's syndrome and muscular dystrophy. A photograph is shown of a mentally handicapped girl whose severe myopia was not noted until she was 16 years of age, although she had attended a resident school (figure 6.1). There is always a danger of a detached retina, and this was the reason for not allowing the myopes in the past to 'strain' their eyes, and for educating them in 'myope saving' classes. Use of the eyes for normal work is not now thought to be a cause of a detachment, but myopes should avoid sudden strains or falls.

Nystagmus is due to lack of visual fixation. If this is due to a

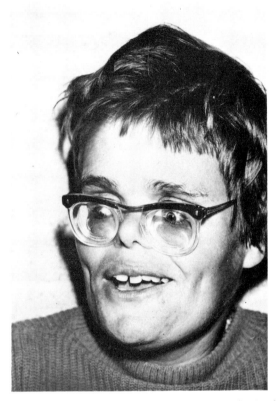

Fig. 6.1 A mentally retarded adolescent girl with high myopia. Her defective sight was not noted until 16 years of age.

macular defect there will be defective vision. In other cases, vision may be normal. Heredity or prematurity may be the cause; but often the aetiology is unknown.

Aniridia, a congenital abnormality of absent iridis, is often associated with a small aphakic lens. Aniridia, associated with Wilm's tumour of the kidney, has been described. It is suggested that in cases of aniridia an intravenous pyelogram should be performed as a routine.

Dislocated lens can occur in Marfan's syndrome, homocystinuria, and as an isolated recessive condition. The lens may shift from its true position, leaving the child aphakic and needing glasses for hypermetropia. At other times the lens may slip back into its correct position, and the child can see normally. No surgery is necessary but he needs special educational consideration.

Field of Vision Defects

These may cause a severe handicap, particularly if the child has only tunnel vision. In all such children, the fields of vision should be tested in each eye. This can be done by direct confrontation methods, with the use of a white ball on a black stick. Sheridan (1969) has shown how the child's visual response to the stimulus can be watched by the examiner through a horizontal slit in a blackboard and an idea can be formed as to how much the child is seeing in the peripheral fields. A child with spina bifida, who superficially appeared to see, was shown by careful examination to have no sight in one eye and tunnel vision in the other.

Additional Handicaps

As with all types of handicapped children, additional handicaps may be associated with a visual one.

Fine (1968) has enumerated these handicaps in 560 partially sighted children (table 6.4). As before, this table does not include children with IQ under 50.

The ratio of children in the intelligence range 50–84, to range 85–114, to range 115+ was 22 : 67 : 11.

Table 6.4   Handicaps in 560 Partially Sighted Children
(Fine 1968)

Handicap	%
Significant physical disability	14·8
Speech and language difficulty	11·9
Epilepsy	5·1
Impaired hearing	4·2
Other defects	8·0
Low intelligence	12·9
Maladjustment	7·3

Regular Check-ups

All children with defective sight should see an ophthalmologist regularly. Ideally he should pay routine visits to the classes for the partially sighted. There is a particular danger of glaucoma developing in cases of aniridia and dislocated lens. Children with congenital buphthalmos may show a deterioration due to a build-up of intra-ocular pressure. Children with retinitis may show an extension of the lesion. Myopic children may develop detached retinae.

EARLY MANAGEMENT

Essentially the mother's problems are the same as with a blind child. Her problems may be increased because the child may take little notice of her and not respond to a smile, and she has not yet realised how severe his visual handicap may be. She must be encouraged in the same way as with a blind child, to talk to him, to put toys in his hands and encourage him to move. Movement of all types, rolling over, crawling, jumping in baby-bouncer, swinging, tricycling and walking, should be encouraged. In this way the child will get a sense of himself in space, will lose his apprehension of the world he only partially sees and will develop an idea of distance and space. He should take part in all the activities of the home, going to the shops and washing up; and his mother should explain each situation to him.

It will be necessary to make the home more orderly. Toys should always be put away in the same place so that he can find them. Doors and drawers must be shut so that he does not bang into them and get hurt. There are grounds for putting padding on sharp corners. The partially seeing child may need a special table of his own near a window, where he can see his own playthings and make collections. A large magnifying glass may be provided on the table, so that he can look through it at objects and at pictures, and later at letters.

Wearing glasses is not usually a problem. Splinter-proof glasses should be prescribed, but it is almost unknown for these and other handicapped children to damage their eyes by breaking their glasses. Albinos require tinted glasses.

Children with this handicap, as with all children with handicapping conditions, benefit from attending a play group or nursery
school at about 3 years of age.

EDUCATION

Partially sighted children will need help if they are to learn; but it is
open to question as to whether education should take place in a
special school, in a special class in a normal school or with the help
of special aids in an ordinary classroom. The presence of additional
handicaps, particularly a low level of intelligence, obviously
influences the choice of schools for a particular child. Some intelligent children with help such as glasses, magnifying aids, a position
in the front of the class and good illumination on the desk, will get
by in ordinary school class. Many of these children with extremely
poor sight are capable of passing examinations and going on to
higher education.

The difficulties that some of these children encounter can be
demonstrated, as glasses are available which illustrate to a normal-
sighted person what the child with each particular degree of this
handicap can see (Kell). They are revealing and help the examiner
to realise the ill-defined misty world in which these children move
about. Many of these children are making tremendous efforts in
competing with normal education. At one time there were myope-
saving classes for children with high myopia. It was felt that by close
work these children stood an increased danger of losing what sight
they had. This has not been proved in practice and it is now felt that
these children can use what sight they have to learn as much as they
can and read as much as they are able. It is also felt that if a child is
losing his sight, due to a retinal or other condition, there is no
advantage in the early teaching of Braille. The child will show no
motivation to learn until sight has actually been lost.

The special classroom for visually handicapped children, which
the Americans aptly call a resource room, must be specially
designed. The room must be well illuminated and the light intensity
on the desk should be of the order of 50 light candles, instead of the
normal 30 light candles. There should be no extremes of light and
dark and the whole of the room should be well illuminated. The
child's desk should be turned away from direct light so that there is

even illumination on the surface. Glossy surfaces should be avoided and the walls, desk and blackboard should have a matt surface. The desk can be specially made with a sloping surface of 45 degrees to help the child to get very near the printed book. He should use a thick black pencil and the books should have large print. As there is a shortage of suitably printed books, some schools have their own printing press for written material and will supply other schools. All aids such as maps and pictures should be large and clear. The child may need to use a typewriter.

Magnifying glasses alone or on stands may be used, but are not always liked by the children. Magnifying glasses attached to glass frames are more popular.

With this type of help, many severely handicapped children have achieved a normal or higher educational level. Many have entered jobs that were at first thought to be closed to them, such as nursing and carpentry. Many have married and their severe visual handicap has become much less of a burden due to early help. In later life, when fewer demands are made on reading and close work, lack of education could be more of a handicap than the handicap itself. These children should lead as normal a life as possible.

REFERENCES

FAYE E F (1970) *The Low Vision Patient.* Grune & Stratton, New York

FINE S (1968) *Blind and Partially Sighted Children.* HMSO, London

FOOTE F M (1956) Classrooms for partially seeing children. *Excep. Child.* **22**, 8, 318–342

KELL J (1966) *Recent Developments in the Education of the Sighted Society. Proc. 1st Int. Conf. Ass. Spec. Educ, London*

KENBY C E (1952) A report on visual handicaps of partially seeing children. *Excep. Child.* **18**, 5, 137–142

MARSHALL G H (1970) *Notes for Parents in the Management of Visually Impaired Children at Home.* Department of Education and Science, London

SHERIDAN M (1969) *Visions Screening Procedures for Very Young and Handicapped Children,* p. 39 Spastics Society & William Heinemann, London

SMITH V H & JAMES F E (1968) *Eyes and Education.* Heinemann, London

VERNON SMITH (1969) *Screening Services for the Early Detection of Visual Handicaps in Aspects of Developmental and Paediatric Ophthalmology,* p. 71 Spastics Society & William Heinemann, London

Chapter 7
The Deaf-Blind Child

This heading covers the group of children with defects of both sight and hearing. Rarely is the dual loss total as in the well-known case of Helen Keller, who, after an illness in infancy, lost both sensory functions, but retained an intelligence above the average. The fact that she had once had sight and hearing had an important bearing on her rehabilitation. This type of handicap is rare today and is not the type that is the present-day problem in deaf-blind units.

Most of these children today have some sight and hearing. The sight may be 3/60 or slightly better; and the hearing loss of the order of 70–90 decibels in both ears.

AETIOLOGY

Children may have the double handicap due to congenital abnormalities. Some cases occurred in the post-thalidomide children. Other children have been born with anophthalmos and absent or rudimentary external and middle ears. In both these cases the inner ear may be intact or amenable to reconstruction, and hearing can be restored to the external passages or the inner ear by reconstructive surgery. It should be considered early to retain the function of hearing.

Congenital syphilis, though rarer today, may cause the double handicap during childhood.

In the condition of retinitis pigmentosa, Usher's syndrome, children with a severe hearing loss may gradually lose their sight due to retinitis in later childhood. The reverse condition can occur, and children with retinitis may lose their hearing. In Refsum's syndrome, defective sight and a hearing loss may be associated with a peripheral neuritis and ataxia.

There are always a few cases where children with the single handicap lose the other sensory function because of an accident or infection.

Postrubella Syndrome

The majority of children in deaf-blind units in developed countries are at present suffering from the postrubella syndrome. These children are usually born at full term but are 'light for dates'. Birth weights under two pounds have been recorded in full-term births. There may be microcephaly. The eyes are usually small, and cataracts are noted soon after birth. In the majority of cases the mother gives a history of rubella in the first 16 weeks of pregnancy, or of having been exposed to the infection, or of having had an ill-defined rash. The chance of a child being born with a major handicap after a rubella infection in early pregnancy is 16–18%. There may be a history that gamma globulin was given, with no benefit, or that an abortion was considered and rejected.

It is important to establish the diagnosis; and this must be done soon after birth. At first rubella antibodies in the mother's and baby's blood are the same. If the abnormality in the child is not due to antenatal infection, the titre will fall off during the next few months and should be repeated at intervals. If the cause is a definite rubella infection, the titre will be high, of the order of 1 : 16, and will remain so. Estimations of the titre in later infancy are not convincing, as the child may have had the rubella infection in its first year or two.

In children who will later have the dual handicap of visual and hearing loss, the visual defect is usually noted first; but these children are likely to have a hearing loss, and should be repeatedly tested in early life. Testing must be done in a well-equipped audiology department. In many cases the hearing loss is profound; but sometimes, when distraction techniques are used, there is evidence that the child has a considerable amount of hearing. The lack of communication and apparent withdrawal may be due to a central communication defect or an auditory imperception. Although the child has some hearing, sounds of all types—voice, a dog barking, plates clattering—have no meaning for him. One hyperactive non-communicating postrubella child was tested in an audiology unit and observed through a one-way screen. He was manipulating a toy, and took no notice of the loud sounds relayed to him. However, it was repeatedly noticed that he would 'still' in his movements when sounds of varying intensities suddenly ceased. His lack of understanding of speech was presumably due to a more fundamental defect than a hearing loss.

Other Defects

Many of these children have additional defects. A congenital heart defect, usually a septal defect, may be present. Surgery should be considered in the same way as with any child born with the single handicap. Some show a form of cerebral palsy. It is usually a generalised rigidity rather than a spasticity of the spastic diplegic type. Epilepsy is fairly common.

Many of these children become very agile. They appear to have abnormal labyrinth reflexes and are just as happy standing on their heads as the right way up. They will fiddle with tasks such as unscrewing a door in that position. Their ability to climb fearlessly to any height and into precarious positions may make their care at home very difficult. Some may be expert climbers before being able to walk independendently.

Behaviour Disorders

These children can become overactive and because of the communication difficulty, withdrawn. The term secondary autism has been used. They may be destructive, frequently breaking windows. There may be an element of attention seeking in this behaviour. They may develop the 'blindisms' of blind children: eye-poking, gyrating and head-banging. The deterioration in behaviour, with persistent screaming attacks, has made some workers wonder if there is an ongoing encephalitis.

Mental Retardation

It must be accepted that in many of these children there is a serious intellectual defect; but with the multiple handicaps, the majority are amenable to some very specific and time-consuming training.

The condition may vary with different epidemics. In schools for the deaf there are some children with a severe hearing loss due to rubella, but no other handicap.

Training and Management of the Postrubella Child

It is difficult to get exact estimates of the number of these children due to irregular epidemics; but in a population of 200,000 there are likely to be 8–10 schoolchildren with this condition, and this number should be sufficient to form a small training unit.

These children may be taken into a residential unit or a hospital for the subnormal, and this may be arranged early, as the family cannot cope with the problem. The child's general behaviour may deteriorate, and as an adolescent he will be confined to a 'refractory' ward having nursing and custodial care only.

Any training which will prevent this unhappy outcome is worth undertaking, although in childhood it is expensive in staffing. Research has been done on the training of these children at Lea Hospital, Birmingham, England (Simon and Southwell) and at the Perkins Institute, Massachusetts, USA.

EARLY TRAINING

Early training must involve the mother and the family. The child has lost what have been called his distance senses—sight and hearing—and must make use of the senses intimately concerned with his own body—touch, smell and taste. For this reason the mother must take the child on to her lap and cuddle him, and encourage him to feel his own body and hers. He must go through the normal stages of motor development and be encouraged to roll over, sit up and walk. All forms of motor activity must be encouraged: baby-bouncers, swings and tricycles. He must also learn the normal childhood activities of clap-hands and pat-a-cake. When he performs any voluntary act it should be rewarded in some way so that he is encouraged to make a communication.

The deaf-blind child is usually not totally deaf or blind, and both senses must be developed to the full. His hearing loss may be as profound as a 90 decibel loss, but at this stage he may learn by a loud voice close to his ear. His sight may be only at the level of 3/60, but he can learn to recognise toys, kick a large ball or try to find a toy that has fallen.

If it can be arranged, these children at a fairly early age should attend a daily nursery where specific training can be given.

Training in Special Unit

The training involves all members of the staff, parents, nurses, teachers, ward domestics and ambulance or car drivers, and it does not consist of teaching the child to perform functions. It consists of noting any response or action coming from him, and working on that. If he shows an interest in feeling materials, his hand is rubbed over other materials so that he feels the difference. The floor of the playroom is made up of different types of surfaces so that he can sense where he is. All attempts at movement are encouraged. As soon as he should be ready for walking he is walked everywhere by holding his hands, so that he gets the idea that he is expected to walk. Physiotherapy may be of help if there is a generalised stiffness, or if the child has lost confidence in walking due to lack of early stimulation. He will show an interest in lights, and this is encouraged by getting him to crawl to lights at the end of a tunnel. He may then learn that by doing a certain action, such as pulling a string, he can make a light come on; and this is an important stage in learning.

He can be encouraged to climb through large holes of different shapes: square, circle, oblong, etc.; and this gives him some idea of shape. His sight will almost certainly allow him some idea of colour and the wall and large toys can be painted in different colours. He thus learns about texture, distance, size, shape and colour.

If he shows any evidence of hearing he should be talked to very close to his ear, and he may gradually develop an idea of the meaning of simple words. It is unlikely that at first he will tolerate a hearing aid. Any babble that he makes should be given some response. It may be possible to reward a babbling sound with something that pleases the child—a sweet or a light going on. In this way he learns that communication by sound is appreciated.

To encourage social training he can be walked to the food trolley, his hand held while he puts the food on his plate with a spoon. He should gradually learn to make distinctions by being allowed to choose. He then goes back to the table and sits correctly. Gradually good table manners can develop. Toilet training can take place in the same way.

Outings of all kinds should be encouraged.

Blindisms can be overcome by keeping the child occupied. If he begins to eye-poke or bang his head, this can be prevented by substituting a pleasant sensation. An electrically operated vibrator, which he loves, can be put in his hand. He will gradually be taught to stop the unpleasant habit.

This is the type of training that takes place in a properly equipped unit to deal with these children. In some cases there may be a real breakthrough, leading to constructive play and learning, but even a little improvement towards social acceptancy is worthwhile.

Other Deaf-Blind Children

With children who have the double handicap and normal intelligence, or who have developed the handicaps during childhood, education in a special unit may take place with a normal curriculum. I have seen a partially deaf-blind child being taught about the equator, with a round-revolving sphere of the world and wearing a hearing aid. Special appliances and a properly equipped classroom will be needed for the double handicap. These children may later communicate by speech or by finger spelling.

REFERENCES

BLIND/DEAF UNIT (1971) *Some Facts and Hints on Management to Parents of Young Children Suffering from Handicaps of Vision and/or Hearing.* Lea Hospital, Bromsgrove, England

Deaf-Blind Children and Their Education (1971) International Conference, Holland, 1968. Rotterdam University Press, Rotterdam

GULDAGER V (1970) *Body Image and the Severely Handicapped Rubella Child.* Perkins Publications, Watertown, Mass.

ROBBINS N (1960) *Educational Beginnings with Deaf-Blind Children.* Perkins Publications, Watertown, Mass.

ROBBINS N (1963) *Speech Beginnings for the Deaf-Blind Child.* Perkins Publications, Watertown, Mass.

ROBBINS N & STENQUIST G (1967) *The Deaf-Blind Rubella Child.* Perkins Publications, Watertown, Mass.

ROYAL NATIONAL INSTITUTE FOR THE BLIND (1965) *Teaching Deaf-Blind Children.* Second Seminar held at Kalundong, Denmark RNIB, London

Chapter 8
Development of the Concept of the Multiple Handicapped Child

INFANTILE CEREBRAL PALSY

In this book little space has been given to the history of the public concern, the education and management of a particular handicap, as this may be of interest to a medical historian only and has little relevance to understanding the clinical condition. This is not true in the case of cerebral palsy. Interest in it has developed almost entirely during the last 25 years and out of an evolving understanding of this condition there has been an increased understanding of other handicapping conditions. In particular out of the study of the cerebral palsied children has come the concept of the multiple handicapped child, of minimal cerebral dysfunction and of developmental paediatrics. Child neurology is now a science in its own right. Children with mental subnormality, speech defects, blindness and deafness have benefited from the 'backlash' of this increased knowledge. The whole concept of the multiply handicapped child rather than the child with a particular handicap has developed from this study of 'brain-damaged' children.

It is proposed to describe the multiple handicaps of the cerebral palsied child in the order in which they have mainly attracted interest.

Definition

Childhood cerebral palsy is an overall term which includes a wide variety of neurological conditions that cause a defect in the child's movement patterns. The World Commission for Cerebral Palsy (1966) adopted this definition:

> Cerebral palsy is a persistent but not unchanging disorder of posture and movement due to a dysfunction of the brain present before its growth and development are completed.

88

Many other features may be part of the picture. The term is not intended to include progressive and deteriorating conditions. It is usually assumed that the insult to the developing brain took place before three years. In this chapter movement defects due to accidents and infections to the brain in later childhood are not included.

The World Commission in 1969 added the following definitions:

Posture: the relative disposition of the parts of the body.

Patterns: that which is recognisable in posture movement or sequences of movement.

Tone: the sustained contraction of living muscle subserving posture and movement.

Stretch reflex: sudden contraction on passive stretching of a muscle.

Spasticity: a persisting increase of the stretch reflexes resulting in a disorder of tone usually with an increased muscular resistance on stretch which characteristically may lessen abruptly.

Athetosis: irrepressible slow writhing movements, the result of imperfectly coordinated activity of the muscles, which are exacerbated by voluntary movements.

Tremor: uncontrolled alternating fine rhythmic movements.

Rigidity: sustained increase in muscular resistance for the duration of passive movement in all directions.

Ataxia: a particular kind of unsteadiness of movement in which patterns are normal per se, but not adjusted to the outside world. There may be associated imperfect balance, incoordination and intention tremor.

Types of Cerebral Palsy

The term cerebral palsy includes widely varying types of movement handicap which are considered in the next chapter.

1 Hemiplegia—congenital and acquired
2 Bilateral hemiplegia
3 Spastic diplegia
4 Athetosis
5 Mixed spasticity and athetosis
6 Rigidity
7 Ataxia
8 The floppy child

Causation

These terms describe the movement defects only and give no indication of aetiology. This may be genetic in origin, due to abnormal development in pregnancy, to an insult to the developing fetus, to traumatic or biochemical damage in the perinatal or immediate postnatal period, or later brain trauma or infection. The aetiology of cerebral palsy is nearly as wide as the aetiology of all conditions in child neurology and will be discussed with each type of movement defect.

MULTIPLE HANDICAPS

As the condition is due to some form of brain pathology there are certain to be other defects apart from the movement handicap. The child may suffer from defects of vision, speech, hearing, language and sensation. Epilepsy is liable to occur. Because of the brain damage there may be learning difficulties and organically based behaviour problems. There may be an intellectual handicap. Emotional disorders are likely to be added to the child's overall disabilities.

Movement Handicap

The condition was originally described by Little, an orthopaedic surgeon. In 1856 he wrote in an obstetric publication on the influence of abnormal parturition, difficult labour, premature birth (many under three pounds) on the mental and physical condition of the child especially in relation to deformities. He stated, 'Treatment based upon physiological and rational therapeutics effects an amelioration surprising to those who have not watched these cases'. Other early writers on this subject were neurologists or neuropathologists who had a chance to study the brain in post mortem cases. Freud (1897) wrote a monograph on 53 children bilaterally affected and noted the incidence of birth abnormalities.

However, the study of the whole child with cerebral palsy mainly took place in special schools for the physically handicapped. In the late 1940s and early 1950s the 'spastic' child took the place of the single handicap child in schools for the physically handicapped.

The number of children suffering from rheumatic heart disease, tuberculosis of bone and joint and osteomyelitis was beginning to decline. About this time parents of cerebral palsied children were making their voices heard and demanding education for their children, who until then had been considered ineducable. As a result cerebral palsied children in special schools for the handicapped occurred in about equal numbers with children suffering from the after-effects of anterior poliomyelitis, with a minority of cases due to other conditions.

Because of the type of children who had attended these schools in the past, the overall care from the medical angle was allotted to orthopaedic surgeons. This meant that emphasis was placed on the movement handicap; and much of the early work involved the study of dysfunction of individual muscles and the resulting abnormal postures and contractures. The treatment was mainly surgical and was aimed at righting the defects in individual muscles and bringing about a correct anatomical alignment. Many surgeons became disappointed with the results of radical early surgery and there was a swing away from this method of treatment.

Phelps (1941) in America was an initiator in the use of calipers, night splints, walking aids and other appliances to help the child and felt that surgery was justified only in a small proportion of children with spasticity.

In England the physiotherapist Mrs Collis advocated a free approach to treatment of these children. She aimed her total approach to organised play and activity. The children were encouraged to move around, swing and ride tricycles. She discusses her method in the *Way of Life for the Handicapped Child*. This method was a breakthrough for children, who up to then had tended to be homebound or hospitalised, and thought ineducable. Mrs. Collis's methods, however, were too free and many children developed contractures of knees and ankles as too little attention has been paid to correct postures. Other writers, Girard (1937) and Egel (1948), had advocated simple home exercises.

Neurological Approach

These early workers had not had the advantage of seeing the cerebral palsied child as a baby or young child. By the time these children were seen in school, fixed deformities had occurred due to the spastic muscles and in many cases contractures of joints had already developed.

The study of the young cerebral palsied child led to a realisation that cerebral palsy must be considered as a neurological defect. Brain damage affects the movements of the whole body. It has been said that the brain knows nothing about individual muscles, but is concerned only with movements.

In the late 1940s and early 1950s a neurologist and physiotherapist partnership, Karl and Bertha Bobath, made a study of the movement defect in cerebral palsy. Bertha Bobath noted the movement and balance difficulties and the abnormal movement patterns, and her husband, by study and observation, suggested neurological explanations for these defects which despite much early disagreement have stood the test of time.

Child neurologists today would agree with the observations of the Bobaths, and many have added further knowledge to the understanding of the cerebral palsied child's abnormal movement patterns. In fact Karl Bobath's explanations were not new. The abnormal reflex patterns which he described had already been noted in brain-damaged adults (Riddoch & Buzzard 1921, Walshe 1923, Kinnear Wilson 1925, and Brain 1927). Normal infantile reflexes had been discussed by Weizz (1935) and Byers (1948).

Abnormal Reflex Pattern in Cerebral Palsy

The Bobaths showed that the cerebral palsied child had retained infantile reflexes, which occur transiently in normal infants and should disappear as cortical control of movement takes over. Reflexes such as the Moro reflex, the asymmetric tonic neck reflex and the positive supporting reflex, which should have disappeared in the early months of life, could still be demonstrated in the much older cerebral palsied child. At the same time reflexes which are normally retained throughout life may not develop or may be prevented from developing by the abnormal retention of infantile reflexes. The head-righting reflex and other body-righting reflexes are retained throughout life. Their absence in a cerebral palsied child was given as an explanation for poor head control and inability to roll over. Balance reactions which are needed before sitting or standing are possible may not have developed.

The Bobaths also showed that a cerebral palsied child tends to be in a total extensor or total flexor pattern, and finds it difficult to adopt a posture that is part extensor and part flexor. In the erect or supine position, the child tends to have the head extended, the back straight, the arms retracted at the shoulder, and the hips extended and adducted with plantar flexion of the feet.

In a sitting position or in a crawling position, the child will flex the head, hips and knees and will show dorsiflexion of the feet. Raising the head into a position of extension while he lies prone causes him to extend the hips, knees and ankles, and to take up a fully extended posture. Another primitive reflex, the tonic neck reflex, may prevent a normal crawl. If the child in an all fours posture raises the head, the hips and knees flex and he goes back into a 'bunny hopping posture'.

A child governed by these abnormal reflex patterns is unable to roll over, crawl or walk in a smooth coordinated manner with alternating flexion and contraction, and cannot walk with reciprocation of the legs.

Reflexes such as an abnormal grasp reflex present in a baby up to three months may be retained in the hands. Alternatively the hands may open in a fully extended position called an avoiding reaction. These abnormal reflex patterns can be given as an explanation of abnormal hand movements.

In their method of treatment the Bobaths have shown that abnormal reflexes can be inhibited and normal patterns of movements can be facilitated. In fact the ability to move normally may be just below the surface. Spasticity, hypotonia, fluctuating tone and the movements in athetosis can be explained as the basis of these strong abnormal reflexes.

Different muscle groups can show spasticity in one posture and not in another. In the supine, extended posture, there may be spasticity in the plantar flexors of the foot; but in total flexion as when crawling on all fours, there may be apparent spasticity in the dorsiflexors of the foot, and the feet may show abnormal dorsiflexion.

This philosophy of cerebral palsy has formed the basis for treatment in many centres throughout the world. Other methods of treatment, such as Temple Fay, Voyta, Rood, are based on a similar understanding of the movement defect. It is obvious that if these methods are to work, the child must be treated early in life; and at the same time as these methods were developing, the importance of early diagnosis was realised.

Early Diagnosis and 'At Risk' Registers

The importance of early notification of any child who was not developing normally was another outcome of this interest in cerebral palsy and 'brain-damaged' children. Sheridan (1960) suggested the types of children who should be specially followed up as they were in danger of developing abnormally, and pioneered the concept of an 'at risk' register. The early lists gave prominence to children born after an abnormal birth. Other genetic and environmental reasons for placement of a child's name on the 'at risk' register were added, particularly conditions which might lead to defects of vision and hearing and to language delay.

Speech Defects

While interested physiotherapists were mastering these new techniques of treatment, speech therapists were also involved in treating cerebral palsied children, many of whom had a motor speech defect. The type of defect is most commonly a spastic or athetoid dysarthria. As the function of speech involves the same muscles as are used for respiration, swallowing and chewing, it is found that these children have difficulties in these essential functions. Respiration is frequently shallow and irregular. Some children tend to speak on inspiration and have a typical breathless speech. The child may have difficulty in swallowing and be a dribbler throughout life. The excessive drooling is partly due to extensor spasm keeping the mouth open. Others have inadequate nasopharyngeal closure. The child may find difficulty in moving the tongue voluntarily. He may have difficulty in chewing. The mouth is often hypersensitive. Attempts to feed the child may cause him to bite involuntarily. Feeding may cause a reflex tongue thrust which pushes the food out of the mouth.

The speech therapist studying these children would realise that if their speech is to be helped, they must have very early training in feeding; and good patterns of swallowing and chewing must be encouraged. In many schools the speech therapist made herself responsible for feeding at the midday meal. One of her main tasks was to prevent mothers and helpers from just pushing the food down a child's open mouth. The chart (figure 8.1), published by the

Fig. 8.1a–h Feeding the cerebral palsied child. How to correlate the feeding to the speech programme; before any child learns to speak he must first learn to chew, suck, blow and swallow.

a Make child use lips to remove food. Place a small amount only on to the spoon. Do not let child use teeth or let the feeder scrape against upper teeth. Give child a chance to bite off pieces of toast etc—do not break off small pieces unless he cannot do so for himself.

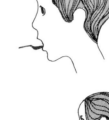

b Have child in good anatomical position. Do not allow the head to tilt back; this will throw all his swallowing mechanisms out of line and may contribute to the formation of permanent deformities.

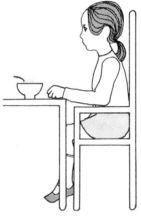

c Tell child to chew and if necessary manipulate his jaw in an up and down motion. Show him how. Vomiting is proof that he is not chewing. Allow him to feel his own throat occasionally, so that he becomes aware of the act of swallowing.

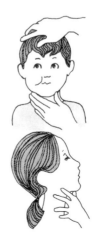

d Place food on one side of mouth, then
on the other. Tell child to move food
around the mouth with his tongue. Do not
place food in centre of mouth.

e Children with speech problems should
learn to drink from a straw. Eliminate as
much jaw action as possible from
drinking—one way to do this is to stand at
the back of the child, cup his jaw firmly in
one hand while you hold the beaker with
the other. If the child drinks from straw
remind him to keep lips closed so liquids
stay in his mouth.

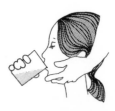

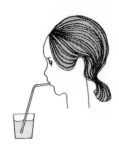

f Children who feed themselves have difficulty in doing so. Keep table-top as clean as possible in order to inspire neatness when he feeds himself or when he is fed by you. All children have pride and can be neat when encouraged.

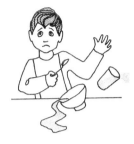

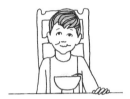

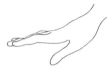

g Praise him when he succeeds. Never scold when food is pushed or falls out of child's mouth. Children cannot help a weak athetoid tongue or overflow from a spastic tongue. Constantly remind him to keep his lips closed and make the tongue work.

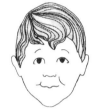

h Always keep dining-room atmosphere pleasant. Direct conversation to children. Do not hurry them; keep confusion at a minimum. When feeding two or more children, feed alternately—a spoonful to one, spoonful to the other and so on. This gives child a chance to chew food properly.

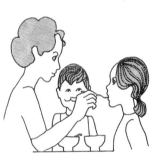

Children's menus are the same as adults. When there is a supper of soup followed by sandwiches, salad, cold meats, etc, very often children are offered only soup, this is wrong. Often children who eat in the dining-room are allowed to miss the soup; only the older and heavier ones should be allowed to do so. Try talking without movement of tongue, lips, throat, the best exercise for movement of these parts are the very acts of eating a good dinner. A good feeder can be the best speech therapist.

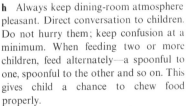

Spastics Society, is on the wall of many units for the cerebral palsied. The speech therapist also found that in treatment they must cooperate with the physiotherapists and adopt postures which prevented abnormal reflex patterns. In many cases, the speech therapist started training normal speech patterns with the child lying on his side on a couch. The normal speech movements achieved were carried over when the child was in a normal sitting posture. With some children it was felt that a pure motor defect did not always account for the child's speech defect. Reflexly the child could move his lips, tongue and palate and the defect was in the nature of a motor apraxia. The child knew what he should do but was unable to carry out the task voluntarily.

Special Schools

The new approach to treatment of the cerebral palsied child made it difficult to incorporate him into a special school with children with other handicaps. Special chairs and appliances were needed and he was removed from the classroom for fairly long periods for therapy. During the 1950s schools orientated to the handicap of cerebral palsy only were opened throughout the world. Many took the child from 3 years of age. The concentration of children with one handicap in a school certainly helped the study of the condition. Two more professions found it easier to use their expertise in helping and studying these children—teachers and psychologists.

Visual Defects

It is obvious on observing a group of cerebral palsied children that a high proportion have visual defects. The most serious, but least common, defects are blindness, partial sight and cataracts. The most obvious are movement defects of the eyes. It was noticed early that these children had a higher than normal incidence of refractive errors. Field of vision defects had been noted as early as 1951, but were not necessarily a serious handicap to the child.

Gardiner (1962) has shown that 34% of all cerebral palsied children have a refractive error. Children with spasticity following a premature birth are liable to be myopic; but for reasons unexplained, hypermetropia—27% is his figure—is common among athetoids. All of these children should have their vision tested early in life. If simple tests such as the Stycar vision test cannot be used because of the severe physical handicap, the child's eyes should be refracted after using a mydriatic.

Eye Movement Defects

The eye movement defects in cerebral palsy are varied, and not always easy to explain. In the majority of cases, the incoordinated eye movements cannot be explained in terms of a refractive error or a third, fourth or sixth nerve palsy. The abnormal movement pattern can only be seen as a part of the total body movement defect—a spasticity or athetosis of eye muscles. In some cases the irregular eye movements improve with use and age.

Some children have difficulty in holding their eyes in a fixed position, and after looking sideways in conjugate deviation the eyes quickly shoot back to the central position. Other children seem to prefer to move their head rather than their eyes; and this partly explains uncontrolled erratic movements of the head and odd postures of head tilt. Guibor (1953) called this spasmus fixus. Athetoids, particularly those following neonatal jaundice, have difficulty in upward gaze. The eyes can move upwards reflexly, but the child is unable to perform the movements voluntarily. This is considered to be due to a lesion in the superior colliculus. The majority of cerebral palsied children have some incoordination of eye movements, and jerky movements can be noted in children quite mildly affected. As a result many of these children do not have binocular vision. Often there is no amblyopia in one eye but an alternating strabismus. The movement defect might affect eye dominance. Cross laterality is common in cerebral palsied children but of doubtful significance.

Perceptual and Visuomotor Difficulties

Teachers in the newly opened special schools for the cerebral palsied noted that these children were experiencing considerable visual difficulties. They had difficulty in scanning a line of print. Some showed a very odd interpretation of their visual world. Some of these children had difficulties in the perception of shape, size and distance, and in visuomotor coordination. Correction of squints and refractive errors did not overcome these difficulties. They were due not to peripheral ocular abnormalities, but to more profound cerebral dysfunction. These difficulties were being noted by observant teachers in many areas in the middle 1950s; and many reported their findings with individual children. Psychologists made detailed studies. The clinicians were informed of these problems by their colleagues in the teaching and psychological fields.

It was noticed in the play of an occasional cerebral palsied child that he could not build up a graduated set of beakers from larger to smaller. He could not distinguish between a large and a small group of objects. He was very late in attempting to undress or dress himself. He had difficulty in getting his vest or trousers the right way round, and the physiotherapists noticed that he did not always realise the position of his limbs. He had extreme difficulties in learning right from left. He might not automatically sense distances in a room; and he would use the sense of feel rather than sight to move from one piece of furniture to the other.

When shown pictures some children had difficulty in making sense of them. They might concentrate on a small object and not appear to comprehend the whole picture. They could not recognise that a man drawn horizontal was a man lying down. Pictures might have no meaning whatever for them. Some preferred the picture upside down. They appeared unable to translate the three dimensions of ordinary life into the two dimensions of a picture. These difficulties could be considered a defect of body image or a defect in perceptual ability. Strauss & Lehtinen (1947) have given the definition of perception as an activity of the mind intermediate between sensation and thought. It is the mental process which gives particular meaning and significance to a given sensation and therefore acts as a preliminary to thinking.

Difficulty may also be shown in writing and drawing. Although verbally of average intelligence the child may be well behind his mental age in copying a circle, cross, square and diamond. In fact children who have achieved reading may never achieve spontaneous writing or copying. Others show their difficulties in drawing. A child may draw a man and put the legs at the top of the page, or draw a house and put the door knob elsewhere on the sheet. These difficulties could be considered visuomotor in nature. Other children have great difficulties in arithmetic.

The cause for these disturbances can be explained in several ways. The children, because of the physical handicap from infancy, have been deprived of moving around and exploring. This may delay learning processes; but it is found that athetoid children show these difficulties less than spastics. Yet athetoids may never have used their hands to explore their bodies or outside objects. The movement defects of the eyes may account for some problems. As the cause of the movement defects themselves may be cortical in origin, it can be presumed that at least part of the visuomotor and perceptual difficulties are due to cerebral dysfunction.

Neurology

Neurologists and psychologists might explain these difficulties differently. Children who can see but cannot turn what they see into meaning may be said to suffer from a *visual agnosia*, as do those who cannot understand pictures. The child who knows what he wants to draw or write and cannot do it may be said to have a visual or visuomotor apraxia. Other difficulties in spatial concepts may be due to a lack of body image and are comparable to the adult cases described by McDonald Critchey in his book *Parietal Lobes*. These children may show right-left disorientation, and Gerstmann's sign. When the hand is covered up they are unable to name the finger touched, although they are beyond the age when this ability should have been mastered. This sign is said to be allied to an arithmetic difficulty.

Research by Psychologists

The field of perceptual difficulties, visuomotor disorders, learning problems and language delay is very much the province of the psychologist. Strauss & Lehtinen (1947) were two early authors who wrote an authoritative book on the subject. Albitiecchia in Paris was using special techniques to help these children in a special school in the 1950s. Her approach aimed at developing a firm sense of a body image. She found that children suffering from the after-effects of anterior poliomyelitis might also show these problems. Caldwell (1956) and Ram (1962) were two teachers who took a particular interest in analysing the difficulties in individual children. Wedell (1960) showed by a carefully controlled study that left hemiplegics experienced more difficulties than right hemiplegics and that spastics had more difficulties than athetoids. Abercrombie and others studied the difficulties in a special school and were impressed with the correlation between these difficulties and eye movement irregularities. Francis-Williams made a study of early diagnosis of a learning difficulty and the way it could be helped in the early years. Frostig in Los Angeles produced a scale which pinpointed the child's area of difficulty and developed a scheme of training based on these findings.

This work, much of which was developed from the study of cerebral palsied children, has now spread to involve the understanding of clumsy children and children with dyslexia and other learning problems. Mentally retarded children are being trained by methods that consider the need to develop a body awareness.

Sensory Loss

On the whole the examination of the sensory defect in cerebral palsy had been neglected while emphasis was being placed on the motor handicap. The study of these fundamental learning difficulties led to a more detailed study of sensory deficits. Children with cerebral palsy do not usually show sensory loss to pain or touch or vibration. Defects in position sense of fingers and toes and in two point discrimination have been noted. Graphaesthexia (ability to recognise numbers drawn on the hand but not seen) may be impaired.

Astereognosis (inability to recognise objects by touch) was noted in a considerable proportion of cases of hemiplegics and in some quadriplegics (Crothers, Paine & Tizard 1954). They could not distinguish objects such as a marble, a penny or cotton wool put in the affected hand. This sensory defect appeared to have little or no relationship with a specific learning problem, finger-agnosia or Gerstmann's sign. Right-left discrimination is defective in a number of spastic children, diplegics and hemiplegics, who show learning problems.

Hearing Defects

It had been realised for some time that some cerebral palsied children had a partial hearing loss. Dunsdon (1951) reports an incidence of 10% in a special school population. Perlstein (1950) reported a high frequency hearing loss in athetoids. Fisch (1955) was one of the first to test severely handicapped cerebral palsied children using the method of conditioning. By repeated periods of testing he was able to show that a proportion of cerebral palsied children had a high frequency loss; and this usually occurred when the condition was due to neonatal jaundice, particularly following rhesus isoimmunisation. It might also follow neonatal asphyxia. Some children with the spastic form of cerebral palsy were affected, but a high frequency loss was particularly noticed in athetoids. It was discovered in children where it had passed unnoticed after periods of diligent teaching in small classes.

A moderately affected athetoid boy was found to have above average ability in arithmetic, but to be two years retarded in reading. It was discovered at 8 years of age that he had a marked high frequency loss, and could not hear the 's' and 'sh' of normal language and did not use them in his own speech. After recognition of his difficulty, provision of a hearing aid and audiometric training, his reading age jumped two years in 6 months and he eventually reached university level in mathematics.

Language Defects

Because of the severe motor speech disorders among the profoundly handicapped children in any school for cerebral palsy, the speech therapist at first concentrated on this aspect of the speech defect. At a later stage, teachers and speech therapists noticed language difficulties. Many cerebral palsied children have a limited vocabulary. They appear to have difficulty in finding the right word. They name objects wrongly. In recounting events they may muddle the sequence of happenings.

One athetoid boy with a high frequency loss learnt to read simple words by the 'look and say' method. He was shown a number of letters on a board and asked to pick out 'Come up, John'. He picked out the three words instantly and correctly. He was then asked to repeat them verbally. He just managed the words 'come' and 'John', but instead of 'up' he gestured the word with his thumb. He could read the word, knew precisely what it meant but could not say it.

The neurologist would define these two problems as an auditory agnosia and an apraxia. In agnosia the child can hear the word but cannot turn the sound into meaning (or has difficulty in doing so). In apraxia the child knows what he wants to say, but cannot say it (or has difficulty in saying it), although there is no defect in the organs of speech. These two facets of language disorder can also be called a receptive aphasia (or dysphasia) and an executive aphasia (or dysphasia).

Epilepsy

Because cerebral palsy is caused by some form of insult to the brain, the incidence of epilepsy is very high. The figures in one survey are given in table 8.1. Children with below average intelligence are more liable to be epileptic.

Table 8.1   Epileptiform Disturbances in Cerebral Palsy

Type	Incidence of Fits (%)
Hemiplegia congenital	36
acquired	61
Diplegia	19
Bilateral hemiplegia	94
Athetosis	22
Ataxia	27
Rigidity	55

For this reason it is suggested that all cerebral palsied children should have a routine EEG examination. All fits should be energetically treated; but there are strong grounds for suggesting that if the EEG shows an indication of future epilepsy, anti-epileptic drugs should be given immediately.

Several surveys on the EEGs in cerebral palsy have been made (Aird & Cohen 1950, Pampliglione 1958, Melin 1962, Woods 1965 and Foley 1966).

ABNORMAL BEHAVIOUR—HYPERACTIVITY

Much has been written about so-called brain-damaged behavior. It has been reported in epileptic and educationally subnormal children. It is particularly noticeable in some mentally severely subnormal children. This type of child may be hyperactive from babyhood;

and due to excessive restlessness he finds it difficult to sit down and stay at one task. There may be a marked inability to concentrate, even when sitting down. Related to this there may be abnormal distractibility. Every change in the environment upsets the child's concentration on the task he is doing. He must jump up and look at each passing car and investigate every sound he hears. Extraneous objects in the classroom prevent him from paying attention to class work. Because of fundamental cerebral dysfunction he is unable to cut out extraneous sounds or sights. This distractibility may interfere with learning in a potentially intelligent child.

These difficulties also occur in cerebral palsied children but their incidence may be exaggerated. One headmistress felt that the child tended to show restlessness and lack of concentration when given a task beyond his abilities, but that when working within his capabilities he could concentrate quite well. The distractability may be associated with a perceptual difficulty in understanding the environment or a visumotor difficulty in performing the task.

MENTAL RETARDATION

After a period of several years of concentrated training of large numbers of the cerebral palsied, it was realised, even when all their difficulties were taken into account, that a number of these children were below average intelligence. Parents of 'spastic' children and voluntary societies had the idea that the word 'spastic' was synonymous with physical handicap and good intelligence; but many are below average ability.

The whole world of mental retardation has benefited from the studies in depth of so-called brain-damaged children. Many mentally handicapped have now been recognised to have the same fundamental difficulties as cerebral palsied children, and out of the work with the latter group methods have been developed to help and train the mentally retarded.

Occupational Therapy

As the children grew older, the need to make them independent in everyday living skills became apparent. A third professional therapist, the occupational therapist, was introduced into the work of cerebral palsy. She took over tasks such as teaching the child to be independent on the toilet, to feed and dress himself, and later to get on buses. Her duties also included the design of appliances. Her advent into the world of handicapped children added a new dimension to the work and made some of the training more realistic. In some centres the occupational therapist trains the young cerebral palsied child in perceptual skills.

Behaviour Disorders and Problems of Adolescence

During these years cerebral palsy became a subject of great interest in the medical, psychological and educational world. So many staff were allocated to help these children in school that behaviour problems did not come to the fore. In fact teachers sometimes reported these children as being 'too good'. It was realised that all handicapped children are at risk psychiatrically. Severe problems, due to frustration and lack of stimulation, were reported by parents whose children were not getting this help.

Some handicapped children have drive, make a good adjustment to their handicap and go on to outside employment. Others, on leaving school, show signs of immaturity. They tend to be demanding of attention and self-centred. They have not been prepared to be independent in an adult world, nor to make satisfactory relationships with the opposite sex. These problems loomed large as the first batch of carefully trained cerebral palsied children left their special schools.

FUTURE EDUCATIONAL POLICY

This feeling of partial dissatisfaction with the results of all the work of the past 25 years has led to a slight change of emphasis. It is felt that these children should do more for themselves. Physiotherapy methods may be too passive for the older child. A method originating in Hungary, the Peto method, which demands active cooperation and concentration, is coming to the fore.

It is felt that the cerebral palsied child may benefit from mixing with children with other handicaps. There is a move to let more of these children attend schools with normal children. In some countries, such as Sweden, special schools for physically handicapped children are being closed and severely handicapped children attend special classes attached to a normal school.

The education for severely handicapped children who are unlikely ever to become self-supporting is coming under review. It may be that the attitude which children have adopted that the only worthwhile goal in life is outside employment will have to be altered. Many must be educated to enjoy life with another eventual purpose.

Chapter 9
Cerebral Palsy—Types of Movement Defect

Cerebral palsy in childhood can be considered as a collection of neurological conditions which cause a movement handicap in a child, due to some type of cerebral pathology. The movement handicaps divide themselves fairly distinctly into different types with varying aetiology, movement defect and differing degrees of additional handicaps. In each type the eventual outcome in the development of skills, in the kind of education possible and in the extent of the handicap in adult life may be different. Each movement handicap is considered separately in this chapter.

Incidence

The overall incidence in different surveys throughout the country varies, but the average incidence is 2 per 1000 live births. This means that in a city of half a million, with 10,000 births a year, there are likely to be about 260 cerebral palsied children of school age between 3 and 16 years. The numbers may be somewhat fewer as some of the very severely handicapped die during childhood.

Table 9.1 Incidence of Different Movement Defects

	Bristol 560 cases (%)	Dundee 240 cases (%)	Edinburgh 208 cases (%)
Infantile hemiplegia	34	37·5	36·1
Bilateral hemiplegia	5	1·3	4·0
Diplegia	33	38·2	38·4
Athetosis or dyskinesia	12	8·4	8·4
Ataxia (including ataxia diplegia)	13	4·6	13·0
Rigidity (other)	3	10·0	0·1
	100·0	100·0	100·0

108

The incidence of each movement defect in various surveys is shown in table 9.1. The figures vary, as different observers see the handicap in different ways, but are fairly comparable.

INFANTILE HEMIPLEGIA

This is the commonest type of infantile cerebral palsy. There are roughly 6 children with this handicap among 10,000 school children.

Movement Handicap

Infantile hemiplegia is a movement defect of one side of the body only, either the right side or the left. The handicap is not always uniform. In the typical spastic form in the older child, the upper limb is held with the arm adducted and internally rotated, the forearm flexed and pronated, the wrists flexed, and the fingers flexed with the thumb pressed into the palm. Unless the child is helped to use the arm, contractures develop in the elbow and wrist flexors and the forearm pronators. The arm becomes fixed and useless in that position.

There is often little abnormality of hip movements, and adductor spasm is not usually noted. There is severe spasticity of the calf muscles, and the foot is held in plantar flexion. Dorsiflexion of the foot is always weak in hemiplegia, unless practised very adequately and from an early age. The spasm in the calf muscles may lead to permanent contractures. Because of poor dorsiflexion the child tends to walk with his heel raised on the affected side, and, to compensate, abducts the hip and swings the lower limb or hyper-extends the knee. Dorsiflexion of the foot is easier to perform with the knee flexed.

In severe cases there is spasm in the trunk muscles of the affected side. This causes a scoliosis, and by raising the pelvis produces an apparent shortening of the lower limb, which in turn causes further plantar flexion. The lower part of the face and tongue may be affected, and there may be an internal strabismus on the affected side.

Associated Movements

In the majority of cases so-called associated movements are present. When the child makes a movement with his non-affected limb, the affected side partially or completely assumes the typical hemiplegic position. Walshe has shown that these associated movements are primitive reflex movements, released because the limb is no longer under cortical control, and are 'postural reactions allied to tonic reflexes and decerebrate rigidity.'

These associated movements must be a serious handicap to the child. One intelligent adult told me that she could hold a cup and saucer in her affected hand, but if she then stirred her tea with a spoon in the non-affected hand, her hemiplegic hand went into spasm and she dropped the cup and saucer. One intelligent boy found that he could not play football by standing on his affected leg and kicking with his normal leg, as the affected leg let him down. He therefore kicked with his affected leg held in a stiff extended position, and gave considerable strain and pain to his abdominal muscles. Work in the gymnasium may therefore be more difficult for these children than at first appears.

Types of Hemiplegia

In a certain number of cases spasticity is severe, and contractures are very liable to occur. At least four other types of hemiplegia are seen.

1 A hemiplegic child may show *hemiathetosis*. There are typical athetoid movements on one side only. In these cases the girth of the affected limb may be increased. Cases may occur where the defect may be predominantly athetoid in the arm, and in the leg spastic.

2 Another group of cases show marked *sensory loss*, with spasticity present often to a minimal extent. The sensory loss takes the form of an astereognosis, and in some cases there is a loss of sense of position. The disorder of motility may be due to apraxia, and not to spasticity.

3 Spasticity is *minimal*, there may be no evidence of astereognosis, and yet the child refuses to use his affected arm. He may attempt very awkwardly to button his clothes with his non-affected hand, making no attempt to help with his affected hand. Yet there appears to be no obvious reason why he should not use it. The child may

have a defective body-image, and may forget about his affected hand.

4   Minimal spasticity and often no sensory loss, but a pronounced *defect in growth.*

Aetiology

The causes of hemiplegia are divided by the time of development into two clearcut types. About two-thirds of the cases of hemiplegia date from birth, and about one-third follow an illness or catastrophe in infancy. There is a higher than normal incidence of first births in cases of congenital hemiplegia.

Table 9.2   Survey of Congenital Hemiplegia: 129 Cases
(Woods)

Genetic abnormality		3
Antenatal abnormality		45
Postmature		16
Delivery:	Vertex	73
	Breech	6
	Forceps	96
	Caesarian	6
	1st twin	4
	2nd twin	5
Birth weight:	2–3 lb	4
	3–4 lb	9
	4–5 lb	11
	5–5$\frac{1}{2}$ lb	8
	5$\frac{1}{2}$–8 lb	70
	8 lb +	27
Neonatal illness		69

The congenital causes (table 9.2) can be described under three headings.

1   Congenital Defects

Sturge-Weber's Syndrome   In this condition there is a naevus on one side of the face, and evidence of a naevoid condition in the brain, causing a hemiplegia of the opposite side. There is usually intracranial calcification. The majority of these children suffer from epilepsy and are also mentally retarded.

Absent Corpus Callosum   This congenital abnormality may cause a hemiplegia. In the one case seen, the child gave a unilateral response to usually bilateral movements. She shrugged one shoulder only, and smiled with one side of her face.

Other developmental abnormalities, such as hydrocephalus, may be associated with hemiplegia.

2   Birth Abnormalities

The majority of children with congenital hemiplegia are born after an abnormal pregnancy or birth process.

Pre-eclampsia, prematurity, postmaturity, or abnormal delivery such as forceps, breech, twin or Caesarian birth may be a factor. In cases where the circumstances at birth were blamed for the hemiplegia, there was evidence that the child was ill in the neonatal period, and cerebral damage was presumed to have occurred.

3   No Apparent Cause

In about 20% of cases no cause can be found for the condition. There may have been unsuspected cerebral involvement during birth, or a cerebrovascular incident as described under acquired hemiplegia.

Acquired Hemiplegia

There are numerous causes for the development of hemiplegia during early life in a previously healthy child.

1   Hemiplegia may follow an attack of childhood infective illness such as pertussis, measles, mumps or chickenpox. Damage may follow an infantile convulsion associated with the illness, or the underlying pathology may be a vascular lesion or encephalitis.

2   Hemiplegia may follow immunisation, the immediate cause being a fit occurring within hours of the injection.

3   It may be due to a cerebral venous thrombosis during pneumonia, meningitis, following surgery such as appendicectomy, and more rarely now, tuberculous meningitis. It can occur after severe dehydration in gastroenteritis.

4   Hemiplegia has followed arterial thrombosis in a congenital heart defect such as Fallot's tetralogy, or in sickle cell anaemia.

5   Possibly the commonest presentation is of sudden onset in a previously well child. He convulses and passes into coma. On recovery he is found to have a permanent hemiplegia. This type of hemiplegia has been the subject of a booklet in the *Little Club* series (Isler 1971). The author produces evidence that the cause of this condition is a vascular anomaly. There may be rupture of an arterial or venous aneurysm, or from an angioma. There may be arterial occlusion due to focal arteritis or arterial or venous thrombosis. There may be trauma to the internal carotid artery. These conditions are revealed by angiography.

6   Occasionally hemiplegia develops slowly and insidiously, and must be part of a deteriorating neurological condition. A cerebral tumour must be considered.

7   Hemiplegia may develop after a prolonged convulsion or status epilepticus in a known epileptic child. The possibility of this catastrophe makes it imperative that at all times active measures are taken to prevent any epileptic fit lasting longer than 15 to 20 minutes.

8   Hemiplegia may follow injury, such as a road accident or baby battering. There may be a subdural haematoma that requires immediate evacuation.

Pathology

The extent of the brain damage in cases of hemiplegia may be revealed by air encephalography. Almost invariably it reveals an enlarged lateral ventricle, and thinning of the cerebral cortex on the opposite side to the hemiplegia. A straight X-ray of skull may show asymmetry of the skull, with a reduced capacity on the side of the affected hemisphere. There may be thickening of the skull on that side. This can be considered a direct result of the damage to the cerebral cortex and subsequent lack of development. If the soft tissue shows delayed growth, the allied bony structure does not develop.

Early Diagnosis

The defect is usually noticed about the sixth month of life or later. There may have been asymmetry in the child's early movements, and persistence of the asymmetric tonic neck reflex to one side. Some parents have noted early clenching of the fist; but in many cases nothing abnormal is seen until cortical control of movement takes over from the infantile reflex patterns. The parents may notice that the child is disinclined to use one hand, and the affected hand may be stiff. The defect in the arms is usually noticed before that of the leg.

Children with hemiplegia may be late in sitting up or in crawling. Often they shuffle on their bottoms rather than crawl. Walking may also be late. The majority of cases are noted in the first year of life; but occasionally a very mild hemiplegia is only noted when another handicap, such as epilepsy or educational subnormality, is being investigated.

Additional Defects

Visual Defects   In about one-third of cases of infantile hemiplegia there is a field of vision defect. It is a homonymous hemianopia affecting the field of vision on the side of the affected limb. It can be revealed by testing with confrontation methods, or by the use of the visual evoked response electroencephalogram. A hemiplegic child with this defect should be placed in a classroom so that his defective field of vision is near the wall, not facing the centre of the classroom. In the majority of cases it is not a severe handicap.

Strabismus, due to a refractive error or to the field of vision defect or to underlying optic atrophy on the affected side, may be present.

Hearing defects are not common.

Sensory Loss   There may be astereognosis of the affected hand. Blindfold, the child may not be able to distinguish a marble, cotton wool or penny in the affected hand, although he can do so readily in the other hand. This blurring of sensation may be a factor in the child's refusal to use his hand. It may be associated with a hypotonic hand and arm in which there is defective growth, rather than a stiff spastic limb. Other hemiplegic children may have a body image defect on the affected side, and this prevents use of the affected hand.

Growth The affected limbs may be thinner and shorter than those on the normal side. This may not be due to lack of use or spasticity but appears to be cerebral in origin. Shortening of the leg may further increase plantar flexion.

Speech The motor control of speech is usually normal in hemiplegia unless there is bilateral involvement of the face and muscles used for speech. This occurs in occasional cases of congenital suprabulbar palsy (see chapter 14). Hemiplegic children may have delayed language development due to mental retardation; but there may be specific dysphasia due to damage to the speech centres in the affected hemisphere.

Epilepsy

Epileptic attacks occur very commonly. The fits may date from birth or occur for the first time in infancy, childhood or adolescence (table 9.3a). There may be frequent fits or an occasional episode. Onset of epilepsy before three years appears to have a poor prognosis for later intelligence (table 9.3b).

Table 9.3 Epilepsy in Hemiplegic Children (Woods)

a Age of onset of fits (in 61 children)

	No.
From birth	39
From 3–4 years	10
From 7–11 years	5
From 11–15 years	7
Total	61

b Intelligence rating (of 141 children—3 too young to be included)

	Normal	Educationally Subnormal	Uneducable	Total
No epilepsy	63	8	6	77
Epilepsy before 3 years	12	11	17	40
Epilepsy after 3 years	14	5	2	21
	89	24	25	138

All hemiplegic children should have an EEG examination. If the EEG record is indicative of epilepsy, small doses of an anticonvulsant, such as phenytoin, should be given as a precaution.

It seems preferable to warn the parents of the likelihood of an occasional fit, as if an unexpected fit occurs there may be considerable family trauma. The parents will then accept the suggested anticonvulsant medication.

All hemiplegic children who have fits should be carefully supervised with repeated EEG examinations. Where the medication is faithfully given over a period of years, the outlook for the eventual cessation of epilepsy is very good. With only a few exceptions, usually in cases of severe mental retardation, has it proved difficult to control the epilepsy.

Intelligence

As an average it can be said that the brain damage associated with infantile hemiplegia depresses the child's intelligence quotient by 20 points. Whereas the intelligence of the normal population can be represented by a Gausserian curve around IQ 100, with a slight increase at the lower end of the scale due to organic mental retardation, the Gausserian curve for hemiplegia is around IQ 80. It was found that the intelligence in left hemiplegia was lower than in right hemiplegias. There is a preponderance of cases of left hemiplegia over right in many hospitals for the severely subnormal, and of right over left in the general population.

Before a prognosis about schooling and employment is given to parents of a hemiplegic child, a psychologist's opinion should always be obtained. A well-mannered, socially acceptable, verbally orientated hemiplegic girl may give an impression of a normal intelligence when her IQ may be between 50 and 70. Entirely erroneous advice may be given to the parents unless the child has had a detailed psychological assessment.

Behaviour Problems

Hemiplegic children show the expected behaviour problems of handicapped children trying to compete with their peers: attention-seeking behaviour, temper tantrums, immaturity and overdependence. The parents need help to deal with these problems. The specific behaviour problems which hemiplegics may show are hyperactivity and sudden unexplained aggressiveness. This is nearly always associated with an abnormal EEG record and with epilepsy. There may be a temporal lobe focus.

Progress

With opportunity and stimulation all hemiplegic children should walk, though the passing of this milestone may be delayed. They should, with training, learn to use the affected hand as a helping hand at table and when opening doors and using machines. The vast majority will talk, the majority at the normal time.

The type of school 116 hemiplegic children attended is shown in table 9.4.

Table 9.4   Placement of 116 Hemiplegic Children (Woods)

Type of School	No. of Cases
Normal	60
Grammar	8
	(expected incidence 11)
School for educationally subnormal children	18
School for physically handicapped children	9
Training School (IQ under 56)	11
Hospital for mental defectives	10
	116

It is not uncommon for a hemiplegic child with an IQ in the normal range at 5 years of age to be recommended for a normal class in school. At the age of 9–10 years it may be reported that the child is unable to read, and is having difficulties in the three R's. This may be due to specific learning problems which do not show up in the early psychological assessment. Wedell (1963) and Gardner (1972) have shown that hemiplegic children may have specific perceptual difficulties; and both workers showed that they were more in evidence in left hemiplegia than right. All hemiplegic children should be watched by an educationist ready to give specific help to the child if it is needed. Cases of acquired hemiplegia appear to have more difficulties than congenital cases.

Adult Placement

The placement of 36 adult hemiplegics is shown in table 9.5. Possibly with more organised early help the results could be better. The majority of hemiplegics with supervision in looking for employment, and possibly some extra training, should be absorbed into open employment.

Table 9.5   Placement of 36 Adult Hemiplegics (Woods)

Adult Provision	No.	Incidence of Fits
Employed	23	1
At home	2	2
Unemployable	2	1
Rehabilitation centre	2	
Provision for mentally subnormal	5	3
Married	1	1
Grammar school	1	
	36	8

BILATERAL HEMIPLEGIA

Movement Handicap

In this movement handicap all four limbs are affected; but the condition tends to be asymmetrical. One side of the body is more affected than the other, and the arms are worse affected than the legs. Usually one arm is less affected than the other. This is partly due to the fact that the child may try to use one hand. Both arms and hands will tend to adopt the typical hemiplegic position of flexion of elbow and wrist and pronation of forearm. The difference between this condition and spastic diplegia or quadriplegia is that there is no adductor spasm in the legs. In fact the non-ambulant child may lie with the lower limbs markedly abducted. The face is likely to be involved. There may be difficulties in chewing and swallowing, and the child may be a severe dribbler.

Aetiology

The aetiology is similar to hemiplegia; but often the perinatal and neonatal illness was more severe, and the child may have had a very low Apgar score or been reported as class D asphyxia at birth. Other cases of bilateral involvement may follow an infective illness, such as measles encephalitis, a cerebrovascular accident or a brain injury.

Early Diagnosis

These severely involved children are known by parents and doctors to have suffered brain damage from birth or after the subsequent cerebral insult. There is usually no period of apparent normality.

Other Defects

As brain damage is severe there is involvement of other sensory functions. It is likely that the child has astereognosis in both hands; but it is usually impossible to test for it. Hearing is usually intact. There are pronounced visual defects, eye movement defects, a field of vision defect, defective vision due to optic atrophy. In some cases the discs appear normal but the pupils react sluggishly to light. The lack of response to visual stimuli is due to cerebral blindness— damage to the occipital cortex. Epilepsy occurs in virtually 100% of cases.

These children are profoundly mentally retarded. There are occasional reports of children who retain normal intelligence. These cases make the neurologist ask where the centres of intelligence are in the brain. The author knew a boy who had bilateral hemiplegia following neonatal meningitis. He had optic atrophy in one eye and a field of vision defect in the other. He had a dysarthria which responded remarkably to speech therapy. There was astereognosis in both hands, but he overcame this by the use of vision. He could do up all his buttons except the top ones. He eventually walked with elbow crutches, and used a tricycle and later a motorised vehicle. His intelligence was normal and he was particularly interested in mathematics.

Management

The majority of these children are cared for at home, in special care units in training schools or in hospitals for the subnormal. There is a considerable death rate in early childhood.

By a supreme effort on the part of physiotherapists and other staff, some of these children have walked and been able to take part in simple play, and later in simple workshop tasks.

SPASTIC DIPLEGIA

This is the original condition described by Little in 1856 (figure 9.1). Many cases follow a premature birth, and this was noted by Little,

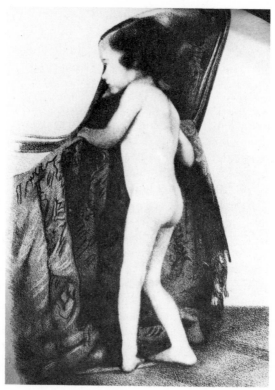

Fig. 9.1   A child with spastic diplegia. The drawing in Little's original article, 1862.

who mentions that many had a birth weight of three pounds or less, showing that some of these children survived over 100 years ago.

The incidence of this condition varies according to the success of methods used to prevent prematurity and of the early care of premature babies. A reduction in cases in recent years has been reported by Davies (1970), and considered to be due to early feeding and the prevention of biochemical imbalance.

Movement Handicap

These children show symmetrical or near symmetrical involvement; and the legs are more involved than the arms. In the erect or supine position the child shows the typical scissor pattern which is associated with this condition. The head and back are held in an extended position, the hips are extended internally rotated and adducted, the knees are extended and the ankles are in the plantar flexion position. It is extremely important, when examining these children, to look at the movement patterns in different postures. If the child is placed in the sitting position, the head may be flexed, the back may assume an infantile totally flexed curve. The hips, knees and ankles may flex, and the child can sit in the tailor position on the base of his spine (figure 9.2). If he is placed prone, his head may rise from the couch, and his body extend with extended hips, knees and plantar flexion of feet. If he is maintained in an all fours crawling position, the head, hips, knees and ankles may flex, and he may show spasm in dorsiflexion rather than in plantar flexion. If the head is raised in this position, the hips and knees may extend. In a less involved child, the primitive tonic neck reflex may take over, and he will acutely flex the hips and move in a symmetric bunny or kangaroo hop.

The increased extensor spasm prevents the child from rolling over, and the absence of body-righting reflexes prevents him from developing a reciprocal flexion and extension of the hips and knees to roll over smoothly. In the same way a smooth crawling pattern is impossible.

The arms may be mildly, moderately or severely affected. If they are entirely normal, the condition can be called a spastic paraplegia. Usually there is some involvement of the upper limbs. If the arms are moderately affected, one hand is better than the other because the child will use one hand for play. The fingers may be spastic and

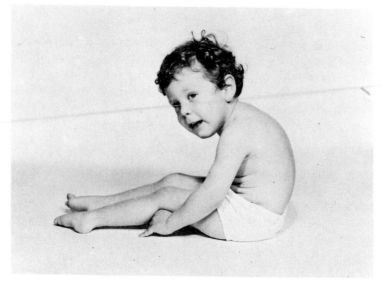

Fig. 9.2 Sitting posture. A child aged 3 years with spastic diplegia.

clenched. In attempting to hold an object, hands may show what might be called an avoiding reaction, and the fingers are hyper-extended. In some children there is marked hyperextension of the first and middle phalangeal joints, but acute flexion of the terminal phalangeal joint.

In more severely involved children the arms are retracted at the shoulders in extension and the child finds difficulty in bringing his arms down to his side when lying supine. Both hands are severely involved and he finds difficulty in feeding himself and playing with toys. If a child with diplegia is maintained in one position for the greater part of the day, particularly if it is a flexed posture, he may develop flexion contractures in muscles and in the capsules of joints. Severe deformities and joint dislocations can result.

In these severe cases the term *spastic quadriplegia* may be used. It is sometimes difficult to distinguish between spastic quadriplegia and bilateral hemiplegia, particularly in the older child when con-tractures and possibly dislocation of the hips have occurred.

Very mild cases of spastic diplegia may involve the legs and feet only. There may be a tendency to walk in plantar flexion only. In some cases the condition appears to be a *monoplegia*.

Aetiology

The factors in 124 cases are shown in table 9.6. Prematurity heads the list as the apparent cause of spastic diplegia. In most cases the baby is premature by dates, and some children are born as much as 12 weeks before they are expected. Many have very low birth weights, under three pounds and some under two pounds. In some cases the child is a twin or one of a triplet. There may be a maternal history of previous miscarriages or premature births, and the birth suggests some form of maternal inadequacy. Other premature births resulting in spastic diplegia have followed antenatal haemorrhages in early pregnancy and also pre-eclampsia. Spastic diplegia may follow a full term abnormal birth, or a breech, Caesarian or forceps delivery. In the majority of cases the child was severely ill in the neonatal period.

Table 9.6 Survey of 124 Cases of Spastic Diplegia (Woods)

Genetic abnormality		15
Antenatal abnormality		61
Postmature		3
Delivery:	Vertex	91
	Breech	10
	Forceps	3
	Caesarian	4
	1st twin	8
	2nd twin	9
Birth weight:	under 2 lb	4
	2–3 lb	18
	3–4 lb	30
	4–5 lb	15
	5–5½ lb	11
	5½–8 lb	32
	8 lb +	14
Neonatal illness		93

There remain two further groups of cases of different aetiology.

Genetic Causation

A form of spastic diplegia, identical to the prematurely born cases, may occur in more than one sibling. Ten families are known to the author. In two families the condition was dominant. In others it appears to be an autosomal recessive spastic diplegia. There is a recessively inherited condition with ichthyosis and mental retardation (Sjögren Larrson disease).

In some diplegic cases there is no abnormality or family history to account for the condition. In these cases there must be a strong likelihood of a recessive condition. The danger of another child being affected is 1 : 4. This type of case must be borne in mind when giving genetic advice. In several cases following a premature or abnormal birth, the incidence of similarly affected members of the family suggested that the birth history was irrelevant.

Congenital anomalies have been noted in association with spastic diplegia. Ingram (1964) mentions talipes, congenital heart defect and congenital dislocation of the hip. The author has seen a case with cleft palate, and another with absent corpus callosum. One child with phenylpyruvic oligophrenia presented as a spastic diplegia.

Spinal Defects

The spastic defect may be due to a defect in the vertebral column in the thoracic region. The condition may be a diastomatomyelia with a bifid spinal cord. A spinal X-ray reveals the abnormality, and should be a routine investigation when only the legs are involved. In two cases seen there was a diurnal and nocturnal urinary incontinence.

Early Diagnosis

Spastic diplegia usually follows an abnormal birth, and in many centres the children are on an 'at risk' register. Many have been carefully followed up and observed. Some cases are not obviously affected in the early months of life. They may show normal walking and placing reflexes in the neonatal period and reciprocal kicking in infancy. The Moro reflex and the asymmetric tonic neck reflex may be longer in evidence than is normal.

The defect is usually noted when the child is late in rolling over and in sitting up. He is late in developing the balance reflexes in sitting, crawling and standing.

Additional Defects

Speech   The more severely involved cases of spastic diplegia show a dysarthria. There is impairment of voluntary movement of the lips, tongue and palate, and the child may dribble. The tongue may be stiff in its movements. Speech is slow and laboured.

Hearing may be affected, particularly if there has been neonatal asphyxia or jaundice of prematurity.

Visual   The majority of these children, even those mildly affected, have incoordination of eye movement. There is typically an internal strabismus, but many children have difficulty in holding their eyes for a period on a desired task. Myopia and cataracts are likely additional handicaps in a prematurely born child.

Perceptual   Prematurely born children in particular show the visuo-motor and perceptual defects described in the previous chapter. Before a child with spastic diplegia is allowed to attend a class with normal children, the possibility of a perceptual defect must be checked. If it is not noted the child may have extreme difficulty with normal class work.

Epilepsy

About a third of the children with spastic diplegia have an epileptic fit once or twice in their childhood, often associated with an infective illness. An EEG, taken as a routine, will pinpoint the likelihood of this occurring. Parents should be warned of it so that they will get help immediately, and the fit will not cause severe family panic. In other cases epilepsy may be more frequent.

Intelligence

The level of intelligence in spastic diplegia has some relationship to the severity of the handicap. A fairly high proportion of the mild cases—possibly 50%—have an intelligence within the normal range; and some have above average ability. Visuomotor and perceptual difficulties occur frequently in this condition, and affect educational achievement. In the more affected cases, where there is severe motor involvement of the hands and additional visual and learning problems, it is impossible to suggest a numerical figure for the intelligence quotient. With individual education they may achieve reading and a high level of general knowledge. The visuo-perceptual problems will prevent an overall good educational attainment. Some are definitely below the level able to benefit from formal education, but there are many surprises. In this group there is an occasional future university graduate.

School Placement and Progress

These children should be diagnosed early and treated as babies on neurological lines. The results of early treatment can be surprising. Eventual independent walking should be achieved in all cases where the use of hands is nearly normal. Other children with more severe involvement of hands should walk with the use of elbow crutches. They may later need to use a wheelchair or motorised vehicle; but enough mobility should be achieved in trunk and leg movements for the older child to get out of his chair independently for everyday living activities. If the child can walk independently early in school life, he should be able to manage in a normal class at school. Others, due to the need for treatment and special chairs and appliances during school life, may need education in a special class.

All spastic diplegic children, whether mildly or severely affected, should have the benefit of an expert psychological assessment at an early age, and early help with difficulties if there is any problem.

Employment

Employment in later life is influenced by the presence of visuo-perceptual difficulties. If the child is physically handicapped and educationally below average, and in addition has difficulties in manipulation, recognising shapes and mastering writing and arith-metic, it may be impossible to find a niche for him. Factory or bench work may be ruled out because of his inability to understand shapes. I have seen a spastic diplegic man using a machine where he had to put an L-shaped object into an L-shaped niche. Each time he approached the task it was an experiment. He could not automatically place the object in position. Visuoperceptual difficulties loom large while he is at school, but may also do so in employment.

ATHETOSIS

Movement Handicap

Athetosis describes a child whose whole body passes into a state of slow, writhing muscular contractions when attempting any voluntary movement. When he is trying to use his hands, his head turns, his face grimaces, his mouth opens, both arms pass into a series of contractions, his trunk squirms, and in many cases he cannot control his leg movements. The abnormal movements in this form of cerebral palsy can be explained only in terms of an abnormal reflex pattern.

The athetoid child may show undue persistence of the Moro reflex and the asymmetric tonic neck reflex. A sudden noise may send him into severe spasm, involving the whole body, and if he is able to stand, he may lose his balance.

All athetoid children, even the mildest case, will show remains of the asymmetric tonic neck reflexes. When the head is turned to one side the jaw arm extends, the skull arm flexes, and in many cases the legs are also involved.

In most athetoids the normal balance reflexes are not present. If the child is pushed over, he cannot put out his hands or abduct his legs to save himself. The ease with which these children are knocked over may give an impression of ataxia, particularly if hypotonia is present.

The tone of the muscles in athetosis may vary from severe spasm to apparent hypotonia, but during any movement spasm can always be found in some muscles and this spasm may pass rapidly from one group of muscles to the other. The tone of all the body musculature is normal during sleep.

Due to strong extensor spasm and the asymmetric tonic neck reflex, an athetoid child may be unable to roll over. He may learn to get around on the floor by using his head as a lever, while supine in an extended position. In the same way he will find crawling very difficult. Some athetoid children have learnt to walk independently, but are unable to roll over in bed or to crawl. Often the use of the legs is better than that of the arms, and some severely affected athetoids have learnt to write, paint and use a typewriter with the feet. Some artists who have done remarkable paintings with their feet are athetoids.

Aetiology

The factors in 71 cases of athetosis are recorded in table 9.7.

Table 9.7   Survey of 71 Cases of Athetosis (Woods)

Antenatal abnormality	29
Abnormal delivery	40
Premature by weight	33
Postmature	6
Neonatal illness (reported)	64
Neonatal asphyxia	46
Neonatal jaundice	24

Athetoid cerebral palsy almost invariably follows an abnormality in the perinatal period, and cases divide themselves into two types—those following neonatal jaundice and those following neonatal hypoxia. The cases following neonatal jaundice may be due to maternal rhesus or ABO incompatibility, or to glucose-6-phosphate dehydrogenase insufficiency. This latter cause is found to be commoner in the Japanese, Chinese and Malayan races. A cause for neonatal jaundice in the past was enthusiastic overdosage with vitamin K to prevent haemorrhagic disease of the newborn. A high proportion of the cases due to neonatal hypoxia follow a premature birth. There is also a higher than normal incidence of twins and of breech, forceps and Caesarian births. In nearly every case of athetosis there is a history of severe neonatal disturbance. There does not appear to be evidence of a genetic or intrauterine developmental factor in athetosis.

Some cases which resemble athetosis, but have not the same abnormal reflex pattern, may follow encephalitis or a period of anoxia in later infancy. Other children found to be suffering from a form of choreoathetoid movement defect may later deteriorate and fall into one of the categories of deteriorating neurological conditions.

Early Diagnosis

In babies who will later turn out to be cases of athetosis, there is almost invariably some concern from the neonatal period. Almost without exception, these children are difficult to feed. They may have been unable to suck, and breast feeding may have been discontinued for that reason. Bottle feeding may also have been difficult; and the mother gives a history of feeding taking an abnormally long time. Chewing and swallowing difficulties lead to problems of weaning on to solid food. In some children, the early difficulties may have been so great that they required tube feeding. Even for a short period this is ominous for later motor speech difficulties.

All athetoid children show delay in head control. The head is unduly floppy. Hypotonia may last for a considerable time, and is

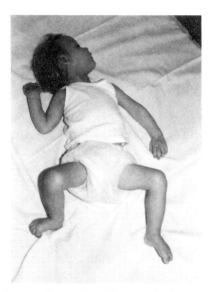

Fig. 9.3 A child aged 15 months with athetosis showing an asymmetric tonic neck reflex.

associated with marked hypotonia of the whole body. Hypotonia lasting into the second year may suggest an amyotonic condition; but usually the abnormal reflex pattern, particularly of the asymmetric tonic reflexes, takes over and fluctuating spasm and tone are found.

In other athetoid children the early poor head control develops fairly rapidly into an extensor spasm. The mother may have difficulty in feeding the child, as whenever she attempts to feed, the child passes into an extensor spasm. Meningitis has been diagnosed erroneously when the child had a superadded pyrexia.

The mother may notice that the athetoid child never sucks his thumb, is unable to feed himself with a biscuit or a spoon, and never puts toys in his mouth. A study of the child shows that this is due to the retention of the asymmetric tonic neck reflex (figure 9.3).

On the whole it is found that the hypotonic athetoid child follows brain pathology due to neonatal jaundice; and the hypertonic athetoid follows brain damage due to neonatal hypoxia.

Additional Handicaps

Speech   All athetoids have a very mild, mild or severe speech defect. It is a dysarthria and may be considered as due to athetosis of the movement of respiration, swallowing, chewing, phonation and voice production.

Hearing   Following neonatal jaundice, and some cases of neonatal hypoxia, there is a strong likelihood of a partial hearing defect which takes the form of a high frequency loss. All these children should have repeated audiometric examinations in a well-equipped audiology unit to eliminate the possibility of this defect, which may at first not be suspected. An athetoid girl of $2\frac{1}{2}$ years of age said to me 'Me walk when me free' (three). Later she was found to have a quite pronounced high frequency loss. With good intelligence and the use of lip reading she successfully masked her disability.

A severe hearing loss may be associated with a mild motor handicap, and vice versa.

The hearing defect is due to damage in the nerve pathways, presumably at the site of the cochlear nuclei. Some athetoid children appear to have more difficulty in understanding than can be accounted for by the hearing loss. There may be an element of auditory imperception (receptive aphasia). The expressive language may be limited in vocabulary, but this can be accounted for by the efforts an intelligent child may make to spare words and make her speech handicap less obvious.

Visual A high incidence of hypermetropia has been noted in athetosis. All children should have an eye refraction examination early. Incoordinated eye movements occur in nearly every child and many have difficulty closing their eyes voluntarily and looking upwards on command.

Epilepsy

This occurs less frequently in athetoid children. If present, it may be of the nature of petit mal attacks. It is presumed that the cerebral defect is at the level of the basal ganglia; and occurrence of true grand mal in these cases suggests additional cerebral cortical involvement.

Intelligence

It cannot be stressed too strongly that these children will very likely have the intelligence that nature intended for them before the cerebral insult. As the cortex is not involved in pure cases of athetosis the child as regards intellectual deficit is, so to speak, 'innocent unless proved guilty'. In fact quite a number of athetoids have a higher intelligence, and have done better educationally, than their siblings. The defect of the inhibitory mechanism which causes the lack of control of movements may in some way liberate the intelligence. It is in this group of cerebral palsy cases that, even when they are severely physically handicapped, there may be high academic successes (figures 9.4 a, b, c).

For this reason all athetoid children should be assessed for education in a school setting, and no decisions made on isolated IQ examinations. Athetoids do not appear to suffer from the visuo-spatial difficulties noted with other groups of cerebral palsy. The incidence of educational subnormality or severe mental subnormality may be comparatively low.

Fig. 9.4 Three athetoid boys who have obtained higher educational qualifications.

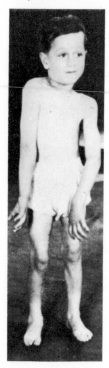 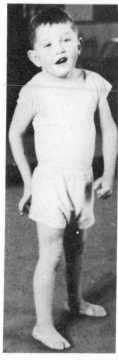 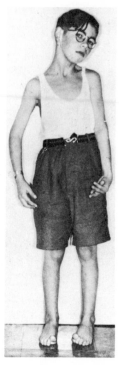

a A boy of 6 years with a high frequency hearing loss, who has obtained a Higher National Certificate.

b A boy of 5 years, who has just obtained a First Class Honours degree in Economics.

c A boy of 11 years, who obtained a degree in Economics.

Management

These children can be diagnosed early, and the services of expert therapists should be available. The value of early treatment in athetosis cannot be overestimated. The physiotherapist can help with the inhibition of abnormal reflex movements and the development of normal patterns. She can help the child to move around earlier than he would without treatment. She can also help with the use of his hands. He will explore his own body and his surroundings earlier if he gets help; and this extra time gained for learning in infancy must affect his later intellectual development.

The speech therapist can help with feeding problems and encourage the development of executive language and inner thought.

If possible these children should attend a nursery school for handicapped children at 3 years of age, so that the various methods of therapy can be coordinated and there can be an ongoing assessment of their intellectual ability.

While treatment continues during school hours, he must be allowed the chances of a normal education. Reading is often achieved at a normal age if individual teaching is given. If he cannot write, gadgets such as magnetic letters or a thick pencil must be provided. Electric typewriters should be available at the time when he should normally be writing. The child's education must include a normal interest in art, music, history, nature study and science.

After help at a special school with education and therapy combined, many of these children may make such progress that they later can take academic examinations such as the British 'O' and 'A' levels. They will need appliances such as the electric typewriter or Possum machine.

Progress for Walking

It was found that about 50% of cases walked before 5 years, and a further 20–25% before 11 years. Some cases achieve independent walking in late adolescence.

Employment

Because of poor hand control, these intelligent cerebral palsied people will not be good workers in workshops or on factory benches. It is a tragedy to see potentially intelligent handicapped people doing the very job they are worst at. Their education should be aimed at more intellectual pursuits such as typewriting, proofreading, computer programming and working the till in a shop.

Because of the severe physical handicaps many athetoids cannot be gainfully employed. If they have educational skills such as reading, they will have much greater insight into their problems and will find it easier to adjust. There have been many surprises, in every case because somebody had the faith to continue with an academic education. Some of these people have shown the maturity to make a happy marriage with another similarly handicapped person. Two have lived together in specially adapted accommodation and managed their own lives. This happy result can actually cost the state less money, as the two together may manage without help at all times of the day.

The whole of this programme depends on early diagnosis of the condition of athetosis, and the determination of staff involved to give them the best environment for full development.

ATAXIA

Under this heading a mixed group of cerebral palsied children are described. In common they show incoordination of movement, defective balance reactions, hypotonia or a mixed hypotonia and rigidity. In a number of cases there is a tremor, often an intention tremor. These children are late in all the motor milestones, and when they learn to walk, may do so on a wide gait with stiff, rigid legs, often showing hyperextension of the knees. Their hand movements are incoordinated and flabby. The percentage of cerebral palsied children included in this group in any of the surveys depends on the bias of the observer. Only a few of these cases come under the heading of a true cerebellar ataxia.

Aetiology

In this ill-defined group of cases there are some where the condition is inherited as an autosomal recessive, and two or more incoordinated children occur in one family. In an occasional family, the condition is dominant and the child has the same neurological abnormality as one of his parents.

The motor handicap may follow a developmental abnormality. Children who survive a repair of an occipital encephalocoele may show a true cerebellar ataxia, as part or whole of the cerebellum may be involved in the defect. In one case of ataxia a post mortem revealed an absent corpus callosum. Several of these children have hydrocephalus due to a congenital abnormality, perinatal brain damage or later cerebral infection.

An abnormal birth with severe neonatal difficulties appears to be a factor in the causation of ataxia, as in other movement defects. Forms of ataxia have followed various forms of meningitis or viral encephalitis.

Early Diagnosis

Children later found to be ataxic are likely to be delayed in all milestones of childhood except, if intelligent, the apparent ability to understand what is said to them. There may be feeding difficulties and late development of speech and of ability to feed themselves. Walking, when established, may be infantile and unstable. These cases can easily be mistaken for children who will grow up to be severely subnormal mentally. The general incoordination masks their potential intelligence. Children of this type may be admitted to a residential placement for the profoundly subnormal before the neurological deficit is diagnosed.

Other Handicaps

Ataxic children may show all the additional handicaps of other cerebral palsied children—incoordinated eye movements, hearing and speech defects, neurological deficits such as astereognosis or a body image defect. Epilepsy may occur. Some of the cerebral palsied children with the most interesting perceptual problems have been ataxic.

These children may have good intelligence, but many are in the educationally subnormal range.

RIGIDITY

Movement Handicap

Some workers in the field of cerebral palsy would deny the existence of this group of cases. The World Commission on Cerebral Palsy felt that the condition did exist and defined it. There are children and adults in institutions for the mentally subnormal who are described as 'spastics' by the staff; but who do not fit into the pattern of spastic diplegia or bilateral hemiplegia. They tend to be generally rigid, with cocontraction of both extensors, and flexion and a type of lead-pipe rigidity when passive movement is attempted.

Some of these children are profoundly subnormal and retain this general stiffness throughout life, lying in a flexed posture with no understanding of the world.

Some children show severe retardation and general stiffness, but with physiotherapy or persistent stimulation the rigidity may be overcome and the child later be able to walk and use his hands. This early rigidity is in marked contrast to the hypotonia shown by some mentally subnormal children.

Aetiology

Abnormalities in the birth process are much less in evidence. In some children the condition is due to a recessive gene, and this may be realised only after the birth of a second affected child, although the first child was born after an abnormal birth—a factor that must have been irrelevant to the condition. Some children are light for dates, suggesting defective development in utero.

There is often evidence of other congenital abnormalities.

HYPOTONIA

In any survey of babies suspected of suffering from cerebral palsy, there will be some who come under the overall heading of hypotonia. The condition has been called one of a 'floppy baby'.

The causes of the condition have been given by Dubowits (1969), and his suggested classification is given in table 9.8.

Possibly the commonest causes of marked hypotonia persisting for a year or two after birth are conditions which will later show defective intelligence. This includes Down's syndrome, metabolic disorders such as phenylketonuria, Lowe's syndrome, and the Pradi–Willi syndrome.

Hypotonia is usually the first sign of athetosis, particularly following neonatal jaundice; but within the first few months of life there is evidence of increased tone in the limbs, due to the asymmetric tonic neck reflexes.

Table 9.8 Suggested Classification of the Floppy Infant (Dubowits 1969)

I Paralytic conditions (weakness with incidental hypotonia)
  1 Proximal spinal muscular atrophies—neurogenic atrophies
    a Infantile spinal muscular atrophy (Werdnig–Hoffmann's disease)
    b Benign variants

  2 Congenital myopathies
    a 'Structural'—central core disease
              nemaline myopathy
              myotubular myopathy
              mitochondrial abnormalities
              miscellaneous
    b Metabolic —glycogenoses

  3 Other neuromuscular disorders
    a Muscular dystrophy—early onset Duchenne dystrophy
    b Congenital muscular dystrophy
    c Dystrophia myotonica
    d Myasthenia gravis
    e Periodic paralysis
    f Polymyositis
    g Peripheral neuropathies

II Non-paralytic conditions (hypotonia without significant weakness)
  1 Disorders of central nervous system
    a Non-specific mental deficiency
    b Hypotonic cerebral palsy, athetosis, ataxia
    c Metabolic disorders: abnormalities of amino acid metabolism
                             abnormalities of mucopolysaccharide metabolism
                             lipidoses
    d Mongolism
    e Birth trauma, intracranial haemorrhage, anoxia

  2 Hypotonia-obesity syndrome (Prader–Willi)

  3 Connective tissue disorders
    Congenital laxity of the ligaments, Marfan's syndrome, Ehlers–Danlos syndrome, osteogenesis imperfecta, arachnodactyly

  4 Metabolic, nutritional, endocrine
    Hypercalcaemia, renal tubular acidosis, rickets, coeliac disease, hypothyroidism

  5 Acute illness
    Infection, dehydration

  6 Miscellaneous
    Congenital heart disease

  7 Benign congenital hypotonia, 'essential hypotonia'

Other conditions, such as Werdnig–Hoffmann's disease and spinal birth injury, call for special investigations.

Children showing marked hypotonia at birth can cause unexpected confusion, as some who appear very abnormal at birth may do surprisingly well and walk little later than is normal. In most cases there is an underlying neurological deficit. Although the child may be apparently normal after the early concern, he may later show neurological deficits and come under the overall heading of 'minimal cerebral dysfunction'.

MIXED CATEGORIES

No attempt has been made to discuss the possible pathological deficit, as this is a subject in its own right. It is known that the majority of cases which come under the heading of cerebral palsy follow some form of birth abnormality. The damage to the brain may be due to many different factors, and may involve different parts of the brain. It can be said that no two cases are exactly alike. It is thus very likely that many cases do not fit neatly into the preceding categories.

A child with apparent typical hemiplegia may have minimal involvement of the other side. A child with a spastic diplegia may show an ataxic element, and some would describe a group of 'ataxic diplegics' (Ingram 1964).

Spasticity and athetosis may be combined. The child may show stiff, typical athetoid movements in the arms, and spasticity in the legs indistinguishable from spastic diplegia.

In some cases no clearcut category can be found for the child's condition. In these cases it is important to make a full description of all the child's neurological deficits and watch the child's development.

Mistaken diagnoses as to category may easily be made. A group of experts seeing the same cerebral palsied child may use a different terminology.

Chapter 10
Management of the
Cerebral Palsied Child

ASSESSMENT

The child with cerebral palsy is a multiple handicapped child. This means that the full assessment of the handicap involves a wide variety of disciplines. Unless care is taken to coordinate the process of assessment, the mother will take the child for numerous outpatient appointments—for assessment of vision and hearing, for investigations such as X-rays and for assessments of the movement, speech and intellectual deficits. There may be little communication between all the specialists involved. The process of assessment needs coordinating and this is best done by a paediatrician or paediatric neurologist, but the emphasis must be on a team approach.

It is preferable if all assessments and investigations can take place in one building such as a Centre for Spastic Children or a purpose-built Assessment Centre. A preliminary assessment of a child may be achieved by three or more well-planned visits to the centre, where one or two investigations are done at each visit. Other centres may prefer to have the child with his parents for a whole day. Centres with home-like accommodation can carry out the investigations with both mother and child resident for a few days. It is impossible to get a full picture of a cerebral palsied child, with all his abilities and disabilities, in one outpatient visit.

Assessment with Treatment

Full assessment is of no use to the child or his parents unless it is a preliminary to a programme of parent guidance and therapy. Ideally the treatment of a young child and the follow-up supervision should be done at the Assessment Centre, which should more accurately be described as an Assessment and Treatment Centre. If the child is attending for treatment, a large part of the assessment can take place when it is most suitable for the child and when he

139

knows the staff well enough to cooperate fully. If the child is attending a centre regularly there can be a genuine ongoing assessment.

Implications of the Handicap

Small babies are amassing knowledge and experience throughout their waking hours from the incoming stimuli received through all the sensory channels—vision, hearing, touch and appreciation of movement. Unless all these sensory channels are intact, and the information received through them is appropriate and stimulating to the child, he is bound to suffer intellectually. If vision or hearing is impaired, a whole avenue of learning is cut off. The same is true about motor experiences. If the child cannot move around and explore at the normal time in his development he will not get an understanding of his own body, or of the position of his body in relation to other objects. He will have missed the early experiences which lead to an understanding of shape, size and distance. Absence of these channels of learning must be a factor in later visuomotor and perceptual difficulties.

Normal vision, smooth coordinated eye movements, stereoscopic vision, hearing in all frequencies and intensities in both ears are needed for full development. Normal development of understanding of speech and of executive speech must be present at the right time in the infant's life if he is to have no language difficulties later.

Anyone responsible for the management of a handicapped child must have this concept of a child's learning if the treatment he prescribes is to have the best effect. This applies to therapists, whether physiotherapists, speech therapists or occupational therapists. It applies also to consultants in physical medicine, orthopaedic surgeons, ophthalmologists, orthoptists and ear, nose and throat surgeons, audiologists, appliance officers and above all paediatricians and teachers of handicapped children. All personnel dealing with handicapped children should have a knowledge of developmental paediatrics.

EARLY TREATMENT

If a child is developing abnormally, and if he is to get full benefit from this type of therapeutic approach to his handicap, he must be referred early for assessment and analysis of any specific delay. With the present widespread use of 'at risk' registers, babies may be suspected of abnormal development in the first months of life. If the paediatrician is satisfied that there is cause for concern, a weekly session with a physiotherapist who understands early development can give the mother some idea of how to help the child. The parents must be sympathetically handled, but if there is true concern they will be worrying already about the child's delayed development, and will be grateful that something active is being done about it.

Treatment well before the age of 1 year has produced good results. If therapy is delayed until 3 years or later, contractures may have commenced which are very difficult to correct.

Therapists

Therapists, whether physiotherapists, occupational therapists or speech therapists, do not usually learn in detail about normal and abnormal child development in their training. To treat young children with cerebral palsy they must have a knowledge of normal development and of primitive infantile reflexes. They must also learn the various methods that promote acquisition of motor skills and help to correct abnormal movement patterns and facilitate normal movements. Therapists from all over the world attend two special courses in London. Courses take place in other areas. All therapists working with children should have access to specialised knowledge in this field.

The therapeutic programme for a cerebral palsied child cannot take place in an adult therapy centre, where the therapist may have to devote her attention to several adults as well as children at the same time. The treatment must take place in a child-orientated surrounding, with the therapist able to give her total concentration to the child. There should be adequate facilities at the Centre for all the therapists to work together and coordinate their methods of treating the child. The mother should be present during treatment.

Methods

We would like every handicapped child to move around, explore his environment, play with toys, sand and water, experiment with paints, and when he is a little older have the chance to join in make-believe play with other children. This cannot always be achieved, but it is the goal that should be kept in mind for each child.

If a cerebral palsied child is to learn to move normally he must be specifically taught to do so. He is a prisoner in his own abnormal reflex patterns, and unless trained to be free of them he may never move normally at all. An athetoid girl may never feel her face or put objects into her mouth unless specifically trained. A spastic diplegic boy will not roll over, crawl or develop trunk movements, unless somebody treats him in a skilled manner. If no treatment whatever is given contractures will develop in the muscle groups and joints involved in the static posture of the child—usually a sitting posture.

Specific methods of treatment are now taught to therapists, and paediatricians, although not experts in carrying out the treatment, must know the principles behind it.

The various methods are described below.

Bobath Method (Neurodevelopmental Treatment)

This term has been applied throughout the world to a method of treatment based on a neurological approach to the child's handicap. It is suggested that the child's movement defect is due to the retention of infantile reflexes which normally disappear in the early months of life. Due to the presence of these abnormal reflexes, normal reflexes which help to control and coordinate movements may not develop. The pattern of treatment is briefly outlined.

An attempt is made to reduce the abnormal tone in muscles by moving the child in reflex inhibiting patterns, without increasing spasticity. The child is gradually taught to take over these movements actively, e.g. a young baby who tends to be in a marked extensor spasm is flexed and rolled over in the normal pattern for a baby, and gradually he takes over and achieves the skill for himself. He has achieved the first stage in a normal developmental sequence and has learnt for the first time the feel of normal movement. In this way the child is taught sitting, crawling, standing and lastly walking. At the same time abnormal reflex patterns are inhibited, such as the tendency to bunny hop with knees and hips flexed and no reciprocation of the legs.

The child must learn normal balance reflexes, which must be present before he will sit, stand or walk. The normal balance reflexes often develop automatically when the abnormal patterns are broken down, e.g. a child with extensor spasticity may try to sit with arms raised, shoulders retracted and elbows flexed. When this pattern is inhibited the arms can come down to the sides and automatically be used for balance in sitting. The child is then on the first stage to being able to sit independently, feed himself and play. Sometimes balance movements have to be specifically taught, e.g. by pushing the standing child forwards and backwards and side to side until he learns to move one leg independently to get a balance.

Often there is a key point from which movements can be facilitated, and by supporting this part a normal movement can be obtained. A stiff spastic baby can be taught to roll over by turning the head, when the body will follow in what is a normal righting reflex pattern. Reciprocal crawling can be taught by moving the head from side to side, when crawling will take place through the legs responding to the head movements. Walking can be facilitated by holding the hips firmly and stabilising the trunk.

As well as inhibiting abnormal patterns, teaching normal movements and normal balance reactions, the therapist must aim at increasing the range of movements that are achieved to reach a near normal span. A child may just be able to crawl, but the distance that each leg moves is so small that crawling is not a useful function. He must gradually learn to make large movements in crawling, and later in walking. Once the spasticity is reduced in hips, knees and ankles, the strength of the muscles and the joint movements can be increased. The child should learn not only to move his knees through a wide range, but to give a good kick to a ball. He must learn to dorsiflex his foot, but also to pull his foot up against resistance from the therapist's hand.

Attention must also be paid to movement of the trunk muscles. A small boy was able to run round in plantar flexion and superficially this appeared to be his only handicap. Yet it was found that he was unable to turn from the prone crawling position to sitting on the floor because of spasticity of the trunk movements. Many everyday movements, such as moving along in the sitting position on a car seat or wiping the anus, may be impossible, even when a child can walk independently and has been thought fit for a normal school.

In many spastic, athetoid and ataxic children this pattern of treatment leads to satisfactory results and a useful independent existence. This is particularly true if the child has had treatment from infancy.

The various postures and movements used to help normal progress from rolling over to crawling, sitting, standing and walking are described and illustrated in *Physical Management of Developmental Disorders* (Ellis 1967). In *Handling the Cerebral Palsied Child* (Finnie 1968) ways of helping the child in daily living activities are illustrated, and diagrams are given of many useful aids to therapy. Techniques suitable for hemiplegic children are shown in the Spastics Society Parents' Handbook, *The Hemiplegic Child* (1964).

Temple Fay Method

This method was introduced by Temple Fay in Philadelphia, America. He looks upon the asymmetric tonic neck reflexes as primitive amphibian patterns of movements. His method differs from the Bobath in that, instead of breaking down the abnormal reflexes, he uses them to facilitate movement in the child. With a child lying prone, extension and abduction of alternate arms can lead to extension and flexion of the legs. Movements in an otherwise stiff child are reflexly produced. This use of an abnormal reflex can lead on to an ability to roll over and crawl; and to a considerable amount of arm and hand control.

Voyta Method

This method, initiated by Voyta, has been used in Czechoslovakia and recently in many European countries. He makes use of primitive reflexes to encourage movement. Voyta describes what he calls 'trigger zones'. These are points on the limbs which, if stimulated, cause the child to move in a reflex pattern which he calls a 'massive facilitation system'. These points are placed distally on the limbs: e.g. when the heel of a young baby in prone is pressed, a massive movement of the whole body takes place. Voyta calls it reflex creeping. He feels that if these massive body movements are created reflexly they will facilitate normal movements in a very young or athetoid child. The method has been found useful by therapists (Levitt), particularly as a method of treating babies, and children in whom a certain diagnosis of cerebral palsy has not yet been made.

Other methods have advocates. Rood (1966) and Knott (1968) use methods to reduce spasticity in muscles, and then to encourage normal movement in the relaxed muscles. Cold and vibration have been used to reduce spasticity.

The Kabat method of Proprioceptive Neuromuscular Facilitation (PNF) aims at increasing the power of a movement by giving the child the kinaesthetic sensation of that movement, and this can reinforce therapeutic postures.

Levitt (1972), while stressing the need of an eclectic approach to treatment of cerebral palsied children, emphasises the importance of a developmental assessment of the child. The child is examined in several postures and his motor abilities in prone, supine, sitting and standing positions are compared with a chart of normal baby skills. The handicapped child's particular delay in motor skills is pinpointed; e.g. it may be found that an older athetoid child with poor head control cannot lift his head in the prone position, which is below a 2 month normal skill, but has some ability to sit in a flexed position, which is a 6–8 months skill. Treatment is then aimed at improving the delayed skills. Methods such as prone lying over a wedge with arms brought forward to play will help the child to develop head control (figure 10.1). A child may be able to raise his head in prone, but can only rest on flexed elbows, which is a 3 months skill. He should learn to support himself on fully extended arms with head raised to a vertical position—a 6 months skill. The importance of shoulder girdle and pelvic girdle stability is stressed,

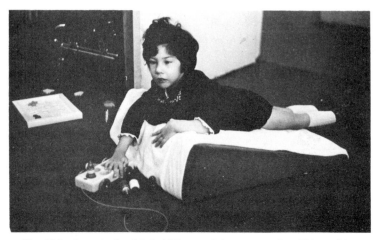

Fig. 10.1   A cerebral palsied child prone-lying on a wedge. This position encourages head control and helps the child to bring her arms forward for play.

and PNF techniques are used to reinforce muscle function. Balance and tilt reactions are taught (figure 10.2). This method dovetails into other methods of treatment, and is a method that can be easily grasped by therapists. It is illustrated in a set of slides by Medcom Famous Teaching in Modern Medicine, New York.

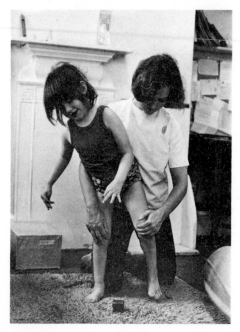

Fig. 10.2 A spastic child learning a normal tilt reaction, which is essential before walking can commence.

Use of Plasters, Calipers and Wheelchairs

Often a normal movement can be achieved by controlling the abnormal movement at one joint. Below knee calipers can control plantar flexion or inversion or eversion of the foot. Their use should only be temporary, and perhaps only for part of the day. There should be a chance for the child to use the learned method of walking without the calipers. Full-length calipers are less useful and should only be used temporarily, to correct a knee flexion or a tendency to rotate the thighs internally. They are cumbersome and prevent the child having the normal experiences of play.

In some children, abnormal postures can be corrected by light polythene splints or reinforced canvas splints, with vertical bands of polythene for strengthening (gaiter splints). They have Velcro fastening and can be put on very quickly during treatment periods, or for activities in the classroom when the child may use an incorrect flexed posture. For older children, long plaster back slabs bandaged to the legs can help to improve stability round the hips.

Where there is an incipient contracture, plaster of paris walking casts can be applied for periods of two to three weeks. While in the plaster casts the child continues physiotherapy, so that he uses normal movements while his abnormal joint flexion is being corrected. Undue plantar flexion or knee flexion can be corrected in this way. A child may wear a plaster cast for about three weeks every few months. He leads a normal school life while wearing the casts, and the eventual result can be excellent.

A collar can be used to promote head control. Thumb splints can be used to abduct the thumbs. Occasionally a form of gaiter splint may be used to help extension of the arms.

These appliances should be light. They should be considered as for temporary therapeutic use only. As far as possible they should not impede the child's play, exploration and schooling.

To give support in standing, young children can be fitted with shoes which have a wide firm base, such as Shoo-Shoos supplied by a Canadian firm.

It may be justifiable to give a young child a tricycle or a wheelchair, provided he does not spend the entire day in it; he can then get around and explore, even though he may later achieve independent or assisted walking. The early use of a wheelchair has been found not to prevent later walking skills. If appropriate, self-propelled chairs should be supplied, and a chair with a one-arm control can be used by children with only one useful arm. Forward placed wheels may help an athetoid child.

The method of physical treatment described are applicable to all types of cerebral palsy. Certain specific points are applicable to particular handicaps.

The Hemiplegic Child

Early treatment of this type of child can be particularly rewarding. Alternatively, neglect to treat can have a disastrous effect on his later life as an adult. The severe deformity seen in some fairly intelligent adults in institutions for the subnormal, where there is a grossly flexed, pronated and useless arm, an ugly gait and severe spasticity of the trunk, can be prevented by early treatment. The child should learn to walk with minimal abnormality and to use his affected hand as an assisting hand for simple tasks.

The child should be helped to use his spastic arm and hand by the encouragement of play which requires two hands, such as catching a large ball. He should sit on the floor on his unaffected buttock and play with toys placed on his unaffected side to overcome spasm in the affected side of the trunk. If he is tilted over he will reflexly open up his spastic hand to save himself. Pushing the child over in a standing position can train balance reactions in each leg and lead to confidence in walking. Temporary use of a plaster cast or a below knee caliper may assist a correct walking pattern while hips and knee movement are controlled. Shortening of the leg should be corrected by raising the sole and heel of the shoe. Without this raise, the child may compensate by increasing the abnormality of his gait.

The Spastic Diplegic Child

In this condition the legs are usually more involved than the arms, and fixed contractures of muscles are more liable to develop. It should be possible to achieve independent walking if the upper extremities are minimally involved, and assisted walking with crutches if the arms are mildly involved. Elbow crutches and sticks can be used as aids to walking if the child has good use of his upper extremities, and has a good sense of his position in space. If one arm is severely involved only minimal mobility may be possible with a stick. However in this group of cases it is shown that independent walking is not the total goal of treatment. If the child, by careful early management, has retained good use of hands and arms, if he has good trunk movements and can get in and out of a chair, and if he has maintained enough mobility to get up and down stairs by holding or crawling, the fact that he gets around in a wheelchair may not necessarily curtail his activities. He can live a normal life and earn his living, provided he has good arm and trunk control, and can manipulate a wheelchair or a motorised vehicle.

The Athetoid Child

The value and purpose of treatment to help these children may be questioned. Certainly many mildly and moderately involved athetoids have achieved independent walking by their own drive and perseverance. Early help and general surveillance may be all that is needed.

Severely involved athetoids will benefit from early treatment. When one sees the mass of uncontrolled movements that a child can show when young, one realises that only the most skilled help will lead to movement control. It is important to allow these children to walk early. Control over their erratic movements will be more difficult as they get older and heavier; and walking should be achieved, if possible, by the age of 7 years.

These children, however mildly involved, will never develop good finger movements. Attempts by parents and teachers to teach neat writing and sewing are doomed to failure. Incoordinated movements must be accepted. Jobs such as tailoring or skilled craft work are not for them.

As some intelligent athetoids may never develop fluent intelligible speech, skill in reading and ability to communicate by a typewriter or some form of communication board is essential. An electric typewriter with an adapted keyboard can be used for school work and in later life (figure 10.3). In adult life, an appliance such as the Possum machine should be available (Jenkin 1967).

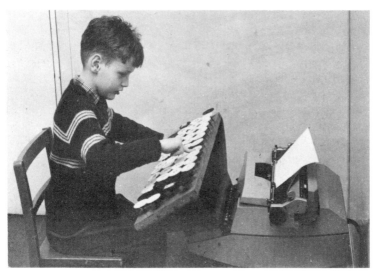

Fig. 10.3 An athetoid child typing with an extended keyboard.

There are many cerebral palsied children who do not fall neatly into the above three categories. Each child must be carefully assessed and treated accordingly. Poor vision may be a factor in poor locomotion. There may be tunnel vision, a severe field of vision defect or inability to see beyond a few feet. In some children balance reactions are abnormally poorly developed, in spite of little alteration in muscle tone, either hypotonia or hypertonia. Spatial difficulties may account for a flexed groping gait.

The Mentally Retarded Cerebral Palsied Child

To obtain the best results intelligent cooperation and drive from the child are needed. The attitude of the mother and family, and the help given towards independence, make a great difference to the end result. It is however possible to help a child who is severely mentally retarded. Usually in these children the diagnosis is made early in life, as the movement delay may be marked. Methods such as those suggested by Voyta and Bobath can be used without early cooperation from the child. Correct postures in lying and sitting are important, even if the child is severely affected. Progress in all normal motor development can be encouraged as suggested by Levitt. Below knee calipers and serial plasters can be used freely to enforce good patterns of walking (figure 10.4).

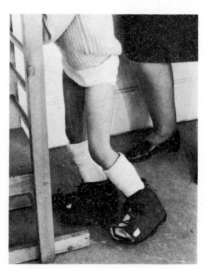

Fig. 10.4 Walking plasters applied temporarily to overcome plantar flexion.

Possibly with these children walking should be encouraged at all costs, without the same emphasis on a good gait as in intelligent children. In later life the mentally retarded cerebral palsied person will not be able to use a motorised vehicle, and may have difficulty in managing a self-propelled wheelchair. If he can walk, however badly, he will be able to get around the home, hostel or institution, where he will eventually live. If he can move about independently life will be much more enjoyable. It is found in institutions that adults of 50 years and over, who learnt in early life to walk with plantar flexion wearing special shoes, did not develop arthritis and painful joints, as was expected.

Treatment in the Absence of Therapist Help

Many paediatricians will be faced with treating a child when no physiotherapy help is available. In some cases an infrequent visit to a distant centre for supervision and advice is possible. The therapist can give the mother advice on handling the child. Booklets and illustrations of how to handle the child can be useful. Many mothers have done very well with this early guidance.

In nurseries or residential homes, where regular periods of individual movement training are not possible, a precept suggested by Scrutton (personal communication) may be followed. 'If it is difficult to arrange treatment for a child, periodic change from one selected posture to another during the day by the use of prone ramps, corner seats, special chairs or standing frames etc. could be very helpful. Any apparatus used in this way needs careful selection and must be made not only to fit the child but his specific needs.' If the child has an extensor thrust, the chair seat must be wedged so that the hips are flexed to less than 90 degrees and maintained in that position with groin straps. A tray or table can be fitted in front, so that he can play with toys. To encourage standing balance, he can stand at a standing table. Abnormal adduction can be prevented by a partition attached to the table, and his feet should be flat on the floor. He should be allowed to roll over and use an infant crawler. The outcome of this type of approach can be rewarding if a watch is made to see that contractures are not developing, and that the abnormalities of movements in athetoid hands are not increasing (figures 5. 6, 7).

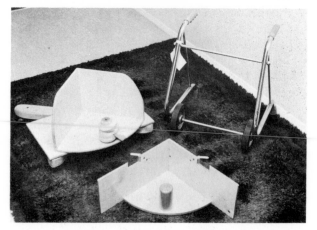

Fig. 10.5 Appliances for cerebral palsied children.
a   A triangular seat with castors to encourage mobility.
b   A rollator to develop early walking skills.
c   A triangular floor seat to encourage head control and
     sitting balance. This can be used with a tray.

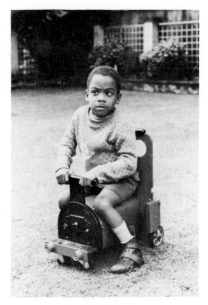

Fig. 10.6   A toy engine to overcome adduction in a spastic diplegic child.

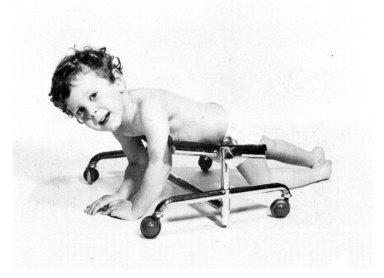

Fig. 10.7 A cerebral palsied boy of 3 years, who by the use of a crawler can explore from room to room.

Results

The training in movement control is the province of the physiotherapist. She is the expert in handling the child. Physiotherapists tend to have their favourite method of treatment, and the majority take something from all the ideas put forward, using what method seems best for the child.

Possibly the role of the paediatrician is to watch progress, and cast a friendly but critical eye over what is being done to the child. To assess progress correctly, there must be an exact record of the child's abilities before he starts treatment, and regular assessments of progress must be made.

A physical ability chart, such as that used at the Centre for Spastic Children, is recommended (table 10.1).

Films are a good method of recording. A routine plan should be followed at each filming, e.g. attempts to roll over, sit up, crawl and walk. If the failure of a child to crawl at one filming is not recorded, the fact that he can crawl later loses its point. Filming should take place regularly, but the length of film should be kept short.

Table 10.1   Physical Ability Chart (from Centre for Spastic Children, Cheyne Walk, London)

Name

Date of Birth

Diagnosis

Approximate developmental age level	*Skill*	*Date*	*Rating*
1 week	Prone—turn head to side		
1 month	Security on plinth*		
8 weeks	Prone—raise head		
12 weeks	Vertical head control		
16 weeks	Prone—raise head well up		
	Prone—forearm support, head and chest raise		
	Supine—engage hands midline		
	Supine—wriggle 3 feet*		
	Get on to knees and elbows		
	Hold elbows-knees position		
20 weeks	Pull to sit—no head lag		
	Sit, lie down—no head lag		
24 weeks	Prone—come up on extended arms		
	Creep—drag lower half*		
	Crawl—hand and knees, bunny hop*		
	Roll over—prone to supine (right)		
	Roll over—prone to supine (left)		
	Supine—lift head off bed		
28 weeks	Supine—lift head well off bed		
	Roll over—supine to prone (right)		
	Roll over—supine to prone (left)		
	Sit—hands forward for support		
	Stand—held by therapist		
32 weeks	Creep forward—amphibian movement		
36 weeks	Hold hands and knees position		
	Prone—get on to hands and knees		
	Sit alone on floor		
	Roll—continuous to right		
	Roll—continuous to left		
	Shuffle on buttocks		

Table 10.1—*Continued*

Approximate developmental age level	Skill	Date	Rating
	Sit on ordinary chair		
	Tailor sitting—no hand support		
	Stand—hold on to furniture		
	Half kneel—hands on floor		
	Half kneel—upright		
	Kneel-sit		
40 weeks	Sit, go to prone		
	Side sit—lean on one hand		
	Prone—get up to side sitting on floor		
	Prone—get up to long sitting		
	Supine—pull up to sitting		
	Pull up to stand from chair, hold on		
	Pull up to stand from floor, hold on		
	Kneel upright, hold on		
44 weeks	Crawl reciprocally		
	Stand, hold on, lift one foot off floor		
48 weeks	Free sit, turn, play using hands (right)		
	Free sit, turn, play using hands (left)		
	Walk—hold two hands		
	Walk sideways—hold furniture		
	Walk—mechanical aid (describe)		
1 year	Crawl—hands and feet		
	Walk—one hand held		
13 months	Stand alone		
1–$1\frac{1}{2}$ years	Walk alone		
$1\frac{1}{4}$–$1\frac{1}{2}$ years	Crawl upstairs		
	Get downstairs alone		
$1\frac{1}{4}$ years	Kneel upright, balance		
	Knee-walk		
$1\frac{1}{2}$ years	Stand up from chair—no support		
	Stand up from floor		
	Stairs, both hands support—ascend		

Continued

Table 10.1—*Continued*

Approximate developmental age level	Skill	Date	Rating
	Stairs, both hands support—descend		
	Seat self on knee-high chair		
	Run		
	Stand—pick up object from floor		
$1\frac{3}{4}$ years	Climb stairs—hold rail, two feet per stair		
2 years	Descend stairs—hold rail, two feet per stair		
$2\frac{1}{2}$ years	Walk backwards		
	Jump		
	Climb stairs—alternate feet, hold one hand		
	Descend stairs—alternate feet, hold one hand		
3 years	Climb stairs—alternate feet, no hold		
	Stand right leg—5 seconds		
	Stand left leg—5 seconds		
	Hop right leg		
	Hop left leg		
	Descend stairs—alternate feet, no hold		

Rating system: 1 = No ability
2 = Partial, laboured, unreliable ability
3 = Reliable ability, but a grossly abnormal performance
4 = Reliable ability but with normal or near normal performance

* Test for independent locomotion, not for training

Note: 'Creeping' is with abdomen on the ground
'Crawling' is on hands and knees

Other centres rely on an accurate description, as in the type of report given below.

Physiotherapy Report

Richard has been seen weekly since mid-May in his home, where the following observations were made:

Head control   The head is held steadily and he lifts it when pulled to sitting. He is also able to lift the head to the midline when the arms are held across the chest.

Sitting   This has improved in the past month, and when placed in *long sit* he tries to balance, using his arms, and maintains the position without assistance for short periods. When he inclines too far forward he is able to correct his position himself when asked to do so.

Cross legged sitting   When placed in this position he can balance, and again uses arms (these are extended and hands fisted) for support.

Side sit   When placed to sit on right or left hip he has difficulty in holding the position (possibly left worse than right) and the legs tend to extend.
Richard is unable to get himself from lying to the sitting position, but with assistance, when pulled up by one hand so that he uses flexion and rotation, he tries to take weight and gain support from the free arm and fisted hand, and helps with the movement.

Rolling   Given assistance with the legs, he can be rolled from prone to supine and supine to prone on either side. He can achieve the movement from side lying to supine, but whenever he moves from prone to supine he 'startles' on landing.

Locomotion   He can gain a little movement when lying supine by digging his heels into the ground and extending trunk and head.

Crawling   When placed on 'all fours' he can balance momentarily, but more weight is taken through the hips and legs, and the hands are held fisted. When movement is attempted, the legs extend and he collapses.
When he is supported with a towel under the trunk, movement is haphazard and the legs extend, the arms inwardly rotate and extend, and the hands remain fisted.

Standing   Richard likes to stand, and gets frustrated if he is not allowed on his feet. When standing with support in his baby walker (a walkie pen type) or leaning forwards against the furniture (sofa or chair) he can achieve quite a good posture, except for his feet and the toes which claw.

Hands Richard reaches out for toys and tries to grasp them. Once he has hold of an object he finds it difficult to release it. The fingers are usually held flexed, but the thumbs are mainly out. He tries using both hands, but possibly he is more successful with the right than the left.

Surgery

The role of surgery in the treatment of cerebral palsy has changed from being the prime method of treatment thirty years ago to the current position where it is used in certain situations only. Surgery may be necessary to correct fixed deformities in an older child, to give minor correction to an older child whose gait can be made more normal, and occasionally to promote normal movement in a severely affected younger child, where severe spasticity in one group of muscles is impeding his mastery of a movement. Occasionally surgery is needed to make nursing easier in an older child where there is gross adduction of the thighs.

To put the limbs into the correct anatomical position will not promote normal movements unless the child has matured to the developmental level for that movement, and the reflexes used to produce a coordinated movement are present. To cut the adductor tendons before the child has developed balance in standing will prevent independent standing. The child cannot then learn tilt reactions which require the use of the adductors. He will not be able to balance on alternate legs when he attempts to walk. Factors such as these are behind many surgical failures.

It should be a firm rule that the child has received prolonged physiotherapy before any surgery is attempted. Surgery may have been considered for an apparent fixed deformity; but with expert physiotherapy it is found several months later that an operation is not necessary. For example, a child with severe adductor spasm may be considered for adductor tenotomy. After therapy, which involves crawling and sitting with abduction, the spasm may be greatly reduced. The predominant posture of the child may have changed from one of extension, as evidenced by the adductor spasm and plantar flexion; and the child may have learnt to walk in a flexed posture, with flexion of knees and ankles. This is a more stable posture from which to obtain balance, but may be cosmetically unattractive. In early adolescence, when the child himself may ask for surgery and will cooperate in intensive therapy, surgery to correct the flexion deformity of the knees may be all that is required. The eventual outcome may be reasonably good.

Elongation of Tendo Achilles

A child who walks, assisted by a walking aid, with marked plantar flexion may invite surgery. Bilateral elongation of tendo Achilles (ETA) may, however, change the child from a position of severe extension to one of severe flexion. Spastic flexion of hips, knees and ankles may develop; and the eventual mobility of the child may be worse than before. An ETA operation may appear to be indicated when a young hemiplegic child persistently walks in equinus. The operation will not remove the spasticity, which is due to an upper motor lesion; in a few years the equinus deformity will return and further surgery will be indicated. It is usually preferable to correct the deformity with physiotherapy, calipers or serial plasters and postpone surgery till adolescence (figures 10.8, 10.9, 10.10).

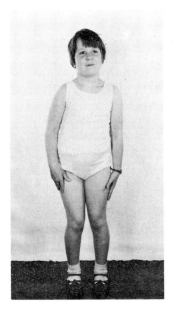

Fig. 10.8 This girl had physiotherapy from 1 year of age. She walked by $6\frac{1}{2}$ years; and achieved a good walking pattern which did not require surgery.

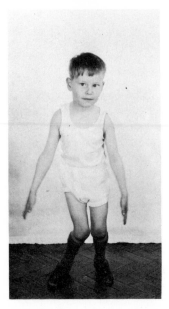

Fig. 10.9 This boy had physiotherapy from 2 years of age. He achieved independent walking when 8 years old by using a flexed posture. Surgery to correct flexion of the knees was performed in early adolescence.

Stabilisation surgery to the feet may be needed in severe cases where walking has been delayed.

Dislocating Hips

One of the serious problems in cerebral palsy, and one which can cause pain in adolescence, is the tendency to subluxation and eventual dislocation of the hip. If this deformity occurs, it is difficult to correct; and the chances of independent walking, with or without surgery, are poor. The hips of any child with spastic diplegia should be X-rayed at intervals. If there is a danger of dislocation, adductor tenotomy may be essential, although this may preclude the chance of later independent walking. Better results have been obtained by treating these children in flexed postures with crawling until the adductor spasm has become less, and a more flexed posture is adopted. At the same time a correct standing posture with flexed feet is encouraged. Dislocation of the hips can be prevented and a

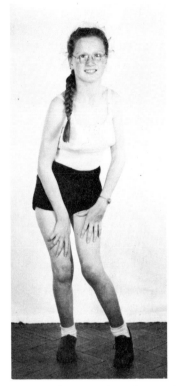

Fig. 10.10 This girl had physiotherapy from 4 years of age. She walked independently with elbow crutches at 10 years of age. She later required surgery to correct the equinus deformity of her left foot. She obtained a university degree.

well-formed acetabulum developed by early treatment, especially early assisted standing in a good posture.

Future Sometimes a child may have progressed well with physiotherapy and attained independent or assisted walking. It may appear as if minor surgery will achieve perfection; and in many cases, as in that of a unilateral elongation of tendo Achilles operation, this may be so. However if the early history of severe involvement and good progress are not obtained, surgical intervention may adversely tip the balance. After a certain time, where a considerable amount of success in a good walking pattern has been obtained, it is best to leave well alone.

The implications of peripheral surgery in a brain-damaged child must be fully understood by the surgeon. It is said that the brain knows nothing about muscles: it only knows about movements. Interference with individual muscles will upset a total movement pattern. If surgery is to improve a function, the child must have the developmental skills and reflexes for that function before surgery is undertaken. In fact it can be said that after prolonged physiotherapy a child must be 'good enough' for surgery. It is not likely to help in severe cases, except to correct fixed deformities and make nursing easier.

Cerebral Surgery

Cerebral surgery has a small place in the treatment of infantile cerebral palsy. Uncontrolled epilepsy in a hemiplegic child may be relieved by removal of the damaged hemisphere. The child must have intelligence within the normal range, as a lowered intelligence may be evidence that, despite a one-sided lesion, both hemispheres are damaged. Results have been variable.

Speech Therapy

The speech therapist's role in cerebral palsy has two distinct parts. Many of these children, particularly the athetoids and severe spastic diplegics, have a movement defect of the muscles used in speech. As the same muscles are used for respiration, chewing and swallowing as are used for phonation and articulation, it is found that all children who later have a dysarthria early had difficulties with sucking, chewing and swallowing. A child who, in the early weeks of life, was unable to swallow and required tube feeding, due to perinatal brain damage, is certain to have a motor speech defect in later life.

The help of a speech therapist should be obtained in the early months of life when there are feeding difficulties. She can help with problems such as reflex tongue thrust, difficulties with swallowing food and saliva, and difficulties with chewing, either by vertical or lateral jaw movements. Later on some of these children have sensitive mouths, as they have never experienced food of different textures. Prolonged dribbling, which can persist during school years, can be helped, particularly if the child is fundamentally intelligent.

Speech therapists working with these children must have a knowledge of abnormal reflex patterns, such as the asymmetric tonic neck reflex and the tendency to extensor spasticity, which causes extension of the head and an open drooling mouth. By cooperation with the physiotherapists, they can work out positions in which to begin treating the children in order to develop good patterns of head and speech movements. Speech can often be trained in side lying at first, and the skills learnt can be carried over into a normal position. The results of speech therapy for dysarthria vary. An athetoid child is unlikely to develop perfect speech and control of the muscles of speech. The speech therapist can feel that she has attained some measure of success if the child's facial appearance has been made more socially acceptable; and the unpleasant grimacing and drooling, which can be seen even in an intelligent athetoid, have been avoided.

The speech therapist's second function is to encourage language. It is no use teaching a child to speak if he has no experience of language. Some of these brain-damaged children have specific receptive and expressive language delays over and above the motor difficulties. With many of these children, language must be specifically taught in the same way as with an aphasic child. It will be the therapist's task to encourage language and conversation between children and with adults.

Some cerebral palsied children, due to the motor difficulty, or to the central communication problem, or to the mental retardation, or to a combination of all these three, may never develop a spoken language. It is then the task of the therapist to find some way in which the child can communicate. It may be by a simple form of gesture, as suggested by Levitt (1969). It may be by some form of communication board, by which the child, having learnt to read a word or understand a picture, can point to his requirements. With the more intelligent but speechless children, it may be by the use of a typewriter.

Occupational Therapy

There is usually a need, in any therapeutic programme, to have a therapist responsible for training in daily living activities. The occupational therapist can give advice to parents on suitable spoons, bowls and cups to help the child to feed himself (figure 10.11). She can also advise them about suitable clothing, and show

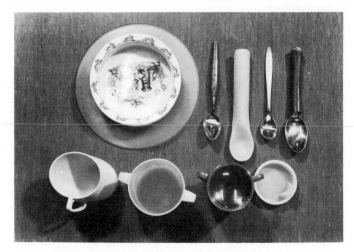

Fig. 10.11   Feeding utensils for the cerebral palsied child.

them how to teach the child to dress himself. In the therapy room, or school situation, the occupational therapist can train the child in a live situation. She can also show him how he can be independent for toileting. With older children she can be the member of the team who teaches independence in crossing roads, going to the shops and getting on buses.

Usually the occupational therapist takes on the overall responsibility of planning and supplying appliances, from bathing equipment and toilet seats to special spoons and wheelchairs. A list of appliances that a cerebral palsied child may need is given in table 10.2.

The occupational therapist is the expert in the training of hand and finger control. She should be well versed in the knowledge of the development of hand and finger control, as described by Rosenbloom (1970), and should note each child's level of attainment in these skills. In adolescence it is often said that a boy will easily be able to get a job as he has 'good hands'. This remark may be made superficially when the actual hand skills have not been fully examined. Many cerebral palsied adolescents have found difficulty in holding down a job because their hand skills were more awkward than was superficially apparent. The occupational therapist should be called in early to assess manual dexterity and give specific help if needed.

Table 10.2 Appliances Needed by Cerebral Palsied Children

Item	Suppliers for the British Market
Wheelchair Baby buggy—a folding pushchair Major buggy—a larger size Tricycle	Department of Health and Social Security
Chair and adaptions Tray for chair Standing box and tray Corner seat and tray Engine seat and tray Watford potty chair	Plans are available in Britain through the Spastics Society, 12 Park Crescent, London, WIN 4EQ
Swedish chairs and tables with adaptable sides and height	Seth Brankell AB, Skanegarten 29, 1251 Gothenburg, Sweden
Children's chairs	Esairan Ltd, Esairan Works, Stevenage, Herts
Car seat—Britax	Spastics Society, 12 Park Crescent, London WIN 4EQ
Foam wedges	Spastics Society
Infant crawler	Carters, Wimpole Street, London Baby Departments
Rollator walking aid	Baby Departments
Safa bath seat	Spastics Society
Suzi bath seat	Spastics Society
Electric toothbrush	Ronson Products Ltd, Leatherhead, Surrey
FEEDING EQUIPMENT Dycem mat—to prevent plate slipping	Spastics Society
Two handled beaker	Spastics Society
Long handled spoons with shallow bowl	Walker & Hall, 22 High Street, Sheffield, SL 2GE
Rubber tubing Rubazote to make a thick handled spoon	Nottingham Handicraft Ltd, Melton Road, West Bridgeford, Nottingham
DRESSING Helmets for protection against falling	Carters, Wimpole Street, London
Dresses with changeable fronts	Spastics Society
TYPEWRITERS IBM + fingerguard	Spastics Society
Jumbo type	Remington, London
Large letter keyboard	Olivetti, London
Possum	63 Mandeville Road, Aylesbury, Bucks

In some areas the occupational therapist helps with visuomotor and perceptual difficulties. The psychologist will have assessed the child on the Frostig or similar scale, and can tell the therapist the type of training required. She may be in a better position to give individual help to children with specific learning difficulties than the teacher, who must devote herself to the whole class.

Dental Care

Generally the oral hygiene of cerebral palsied children is poor. This may be due to several factors. Because of poor muscular control and difficulty in swallowing, particles of food may adhere to the teeth. Due to a premature birth or neonatal jaundice there may be enamel hypoplasia. Because of a tongue thrust or a hypersensitive mouth, it may be difficult to clean the teeth. Malocclusion is a common occurrence.

As these children, particularly the athetoids, may never be able to wear dentures, and absent teeth may increase the speech problems, it is important that they receive good conservative dental care.

To give dental treatment to severely handicapped children, extra time and special facilities are needed in the dental surgery. The child can sit on a tipped chair with adequate head support, but often it is better if an adult takes the child on her lap. No glass mirrors or appliances should be put in the mouth, as they may cause a reflex closure of the jaw and damage to instruments and child. A gag must be expertly introduced first. With patience and extra staff nearly all dental procedures can be carried out without an anaesthetic. Orthodontic care should also be given.

As it is important to prevent dental caries fluoride tablets can be given to the child, and a battery operated toothbrush may be helpful for cleaning.

Use of Drugs

Drugs have a limited use in the treatment of cerebral palsy and come under three headings:

1 If the cerebral palsied child is an epileptic, he should be treated pharmaceutically in exactly the same way as a non-handicapped epileptic child. Possibly phenytoin should be avoided in a child with

poor balance reactions. Mysoline occasionally causes severe loss of tone in an athetoid, and may render him non-mobile.

2 Tranquillizers have a place with an overactive child, and also with an apprehensive child who is resisting treatment. Temporary use of chlorpromazine, thioridazine, chlordiazepoxide or diazepam has been useful.

3 Many drugs have been tried out as muscle relaxants, with very disappointing results. Diazepam and chlordiazepoxide may be of some benefit. Carisoprodol has not lived up to its early expectations. Small doses of mysoline, 10 to 25 mg two or three times a day, have occasionally helped a very stiff athetoid.

It is felt that a drug that will help spasticity and athetosis may be 'just round the corner'. Paediatricians and doctors treating these children have a certain responsibility to try out promising drugs, if there is a likelihood of benefit.

Schooling

As these children are multiply handicapped, normal classroom education is not appropriate, particularly in the early years.

It is hoped that many cerebral palsied children will have had early treatment, and by the age of 3 years they will have some form of mobility in rolling, crawling or walking. They should have experienced normal play activities with water and sand, and have some form of communication. But there will be intelligent children who have not made this progress.

At 3 years of age these children require a 'playgroup' or 'nursery school' type of provision even more than normal children, as they are likely to have missed out on many childhood experiences. It can be argued with equal force that the handicapped child should be educated with normal children or with other handicapped children. If he is in a group of active normal children, there must be good supervision to make sure that he is taking part in all possible play activities, and is not being merely 'babied' by other children. An additional member of staff may be needed, if there are several handicapped children in a normal playgroup.

At a later age these children must have a chance to learn normal educational skills. Many severely handicapped children can learn to read at a normal age. This has been possible in severely involved athetoid children, and at a somewhat later age in severely deaf athetoids. Short individual teaching periods may achieve better results than teaching in classes, particularly if the child has special learning and visuomotor difficulties. The child may need appliances to help with writing. Thick handled pencils, magnetic letters and numbers, and electric typewriters may be needed. An athetoid child with very poor use of hands may need to type with a stick attached to a head piece. Ordinary education should go ahead, with opportunities for creative activities such as art and music and modified

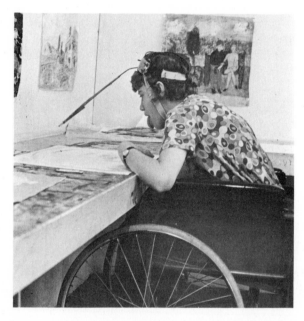

Fig. 10.12 An athetoid girl, painting with the use of a unicorn head appliance. This girl learnt to read at 5 years of age, despite a severe handicap.

sporting activities (figure 10.12). Where normal games are not of any advantage, periods of play and activity in a specially designed adventure playground can fill the gap.

Mentally retarded children can join in the type of training that is given to non-handicapped children of the same intelligence level.

Therapy

In nursery school and normal school, therapy must continue. The child's day may be very broken up with attendance for physiotherapy, speech therapy and perhaps occupational therapy. There must also be arrangements to give help to children with visual and hearing defects. This demands careful and friendly cooperation between teachers and therapists, particularly as therapists will need to supervise the chairs the children use, and the postures they take up in the classroom. For this reason it is felt, in some areas, that schools designed for cerebral palsied children alone give them more help, and that specific help cannot be given so easily if they are expected to mix with children with a wide variety of handicaps in a school for physically handicapped children. This is open to question.

Peto Method

To obviate the difficulty of so many people handling the cerebral palsied child, a method of looking after him which was devised by the late Professor Peto in Hungary is gaining popularity. In that country children are treated by one person only, called a conductor. She has had a basic training in the therapies and in education, but the total approach is a unique one. Children are encouraged to carry out all movements themselves without handling by the therapist. They vocalise their activities so that speech is encouraged, and they develop a sense of body image and awareness of their activities. They are encouraged to develop all normal activities by first getting mastery over essential movements. This is intended to encourage independence and problem solving. Some handicapped children have developed more independence and sense of achievement by this method than by more passive treatment. It is essentially an educational method which takes place in groups or classes, and in its purest form is carried out throughout the whole day (figure 10.13).

An imitation of this method can be used with small groups of similarly handicapped children, who can progress together to develop everyday skills (figure 10.14).

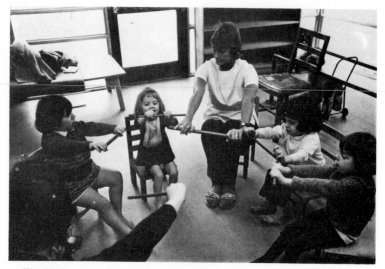

Fig. 10.13 A group method of treatment, based on the Peto method. Note the chairs, adapted for the individual child.

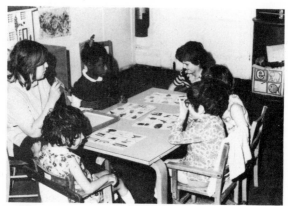

Fig. 10.14 A class of mentally retarded cerebral palsied children.

REFERENCES

ABERCROMBIE M L J (1960) Perception and eye movements. *Cerebral Palsy Bull.* **2**, 3

ABERCROMBIE M L J (1964) *Perceptual and Visuomotor Disorder in Cerebral Palsy—a Review of the Literature.* Heinemann, London

ALBITRECCIA S I (1958) Recognition and treatment of disturbances of the body image. *Cerebral Palsy Bull.* **1**, 4, 12

ALEXANDER G L & NORMAN R M (1966) *Sturge Weber Syndrome.* John Wright, Bristol

BLENCOWE S ed. (1969) *Cerebral Palsy and the Young Child.* Livingstone, London

BOBATH (1966) *The Motor Deficit in Patients with Cerebral Palsy.* Clinics in Developmental Medicine, No. 23. Spastics Society & William Heinemann, London

BOBATH (1967) The very early treatment of cerebral palsy. *Dev. Med. Childh. Neurol.* **94**, 373

BRAIN R W (1955) *Neurology*, Vol. 3. Butterworth, London

BYERS R K (1941) Tonic reflexes in children. *Amer. J. Dis. Child.* **61**, 915

CASS M (1965) *Speech Habilitation in Cerebral Palsy.* Hafner, New York

COLLIS E (1947) *Way of Life for the Handicapped Child.* Faber & Faber, London

COLLIS E (1954) Some differential characteristics of cerebral motor defects in infancy. *Arch. Dis. Childh.* **29**, 144

COTON E (1967) From Hungary, the Peto method. *Spec. Educ.* **56**, 4

COTON E (1970) *Integration of Treatment and Education in Cerebral Palsy.* Physiotherapy, London

CRITCHLEY M (1953) *Parietal Lobes.* Arnold, London

CULLOTY N V (1964) *The Hemiplegic Child.* Parents' Handbook No. 5. Spastics Society, London

DENHOFF E (1963) *Drugs in Cerebral Palsy. Clinics in Developmental Medicine*, No. 16. Spastics Society & William Heinemann, London

DUBOWITZ (1969) *The Floppy Infant. Clinics in Developmental Medicine* No. 31. Spastics Society & William Heinemann, London

DUNSDON M (1951) *The Educability of Cerebral Palsied Children.* Newns, London

EGEL P I (1948) *Technique of Treatment for the Cerebral Palsied Child.* Mosby, St Louis

ELLIS E (1967) *The Physical Management of Developmental Disorders. Clinics in Developmental Medicine*, No. 26. Spastics Society & William Heinemann, London

FAY TEMPLE (1955) The origin of human movement. *Town Psychiat.* **3**, 144

FINNIE N (1968) *Handling the Young Cerebral Palsied Child at Home.* Heinemann, London

FISCH L (1955) Deafness in cerebral palsied school children. *Lancet*, **2**, 370

FOLEY J (1968) Deterioration in the E.E.G. in children with cerebral palsy. *Dev. Med.* **10**, 3

FRANCIS WILLIAMS J (1970) *Children with Specific Learning Difficulties.* Pergamon, Oxford

FREUD S (1897) *Infantile Cerebral Palsy*, ed. Nothangel, Vol. 9, p. 6. Vienna

FROSTIG M, LEFEVER D W & WHITTLESEY J R B (1961) *A Development Test of Visual Perception.* College of Special Education, London

GARDNER L (1961) *Some Educational and Psychological Problems Associated with Hemiplegia. Clinics in Developmental Medicine, No. 4.* Spastics Society & William Heinemann, London

GERSTMANN T (1940) Syndrome of finger agnosia, disorientation for right and left, agraphia and acalculia. *Arch. Neurol. Psychiat.* **44**, 398

GIRARD P M (1937) *Home Treatment of Spastic Paralysis,* Lippincott, Philadelphia.

GUIBOR C P (1953) Eye defects in cerebral palsy. *Amer. J. phys. Med.* **32**, 342

HENDERSON J (1961) *Cerebral Palsy in Childhood and Adolescence.* Livingstone, London

HOLT K S (1967) *Assessment of Cerebral Palsy, Vol. 1. Motor Function.* Lloyd Luke, London

HOLT K S & REYNELL J K *Assessment of Cerebral Palsy, Vol. 2. Speech and Psychological Function.* Lloyd Luke, London

INGRAM T T S (1962) Congenital ataxic syndromes in cerebral palsy. *Acta paediat.* **51**, 209

INGRAM T T S (1964) *Paediatric Aspects of Cerebral Palsy.* Livingstone, London

JENKIN R (1967) Possum. A new communication aid. *Spec. Educ.* **56**, 1

KINNIER WILSON S (1925) Some disorders of motility and muscle tone. *Neurology,* **2**, 891. Butterworth, London

KNOTT M & VOSS D E (1969) *Proprioceptive Neuromuscular Facilitation.* Hoeber & Harper, New York

LE GAY BRERETON B (1972) *Basic Abilities.* Spastics Centre, New South Wales, Australia

LEVITT S (1969) *On the Treatment of Spastic Pareses. Proc. Neurol. Rehab, Stockholm*

LEVITT S (1970) *Adaptation of PNF in Cerebral Palsy. Proc. World Confed. for Physical Therapy Congress, Amsterdam*

LITTLE W J (1853) *On Deformities.* Longman, London

LORING J ed. (1968) *Assessment of the Cerebral Palsied Child.* Heinemann, London

McGRAW S (1942) *The Neuro-Muscular Maturation of the Human Infant.* Columbia University Press, New York

McKISSOCK W (1953) Infantile hemiplegia. *Proc. roy. Soc. Med.* **46**, 431

MILANI-COMPARETTI A (1967) Routine developmental examination in normal and retarded children. *Dev. Med. Childh. Neurol.* **9**

MONFRAIX C & TARDIEU G (1961) Development of manual perception in the child with cerebral palsy during reeducation. *Cerebral Palsy Bull.* **3**, 6

MOORE G (1971) *Teaching a Handicapped Child to Dress.* Spastics Society, London

PAINE R S (1964) The evolution of infantile postural reflexes in the presence of chronic brain syndromes. *Dev. Med. Childh. Neurol.* **6**, 345

PHELPS W M (1948) Characteristic variations in cerebral palsy. *Nerv. Chd* **7**, 10

RAM M J (1960) *The Education of a Child in a Special School for Cerebral Palsy.* British Council for the Welfare of Spastics, London

RAM M J (1962) Some educational aspects of the visuo-spatial handicap in cerebral palsied children. *Spast. Quart.* **11**, 1

RIDDOCH G & BUZZARD E F (1921) Reflex movements and postural reactions in quadriplegics and hemiplegics. *Brain,* **44**, 464

ROSENBLOOM L & HORTON M E (1970) The maturation of fine prehension in young children. *Dev. Med. Childh. Neurol.* **13**, 1, 3

SHERRINGTON C S (1923) *The Integrative Action of the Nervous System.* Constable, London

STRAUSS A A & LEHTINEN L E (1955) *Psychopathology and Education of the Brain Injured Child.* Grune & Stratton, New York

SWALLOW J N (1966) The dental care of the physically handicapped child. *British dent. J.* **120**, 35

TIZARD J P M, PAINE R S & GOTHERS B (1954) Disturbance of sensation in children with hemiplegia. *J. Amer. med. Ass.* **155**, 628

VERNON SMITH (1969) *Aspects of Developmental and Paediatric Ophthalmology.* Heinemann, London

VOYTA V (1966) Reflex creeping as a rehabilitation programme. *Cs. Neurol.* (*Czech*) **29**, 234

WALSHE F M R (1923) On certain tonic or postural reflexes in hemiplegia. *Brain,* **46**, 2

WEDELL K (1961) *Study of Perceptual Ability in Children with Hemiplegia. Clinics in Developmental Medicine,* No. 4. Spastics Society & William Heinemann, London

WEDELL K (1966) The visual perception of cerebral palsied children. *Child Psychol. Psychiat.* **1**, 215

WESTLAKE H & RUTHERFORD D (1961) *Speech Therapy for the Cerebral Palsied.* National Society for Crippled children and Adults, Illinois

WEYMAN J (1971) *The Dental Care of Handicapped Children.* Churchill, London

WOODS G E (1957) *Cerebral Palsy in Childhood.* Wright, Bristol

WOODS G E (1963) Some observations on 141 cases of infantile hemiplegia. *Cerebral Palsy Rev.* **24**, 11

WOODS G E (1964) The outcome of physical treatment in cerebral palsy. *Cerebral Palsy Rev.* **25**, 5

WOODS G E (1965) Some clinical notes and E.E.G. findings in cerebral palsy. *Arch. Dis. Childh.* **40**, 212

Chapter 11
Mental Retardation or Mental Deficiency

The term 'mental defective' has been used to classify a child or an adult whose intelligence quotient is under 50. In everyday usage the term describes the child who, at all levels of development and maturation, in motor skills, in daily living activities, in language development and in understanding and appreciation of situations, has the abilities of a child less than half his actual age.

Under the Mental Health Act (1959) in Britain, this group has been designated mentally severely subnormal, and children with IQ 50–70 have been called mentally subnormal. These terms, like the terms mental defective, imbecile and idiot, have developed an unpleasant connotation. It is proposed to use the description mental retardation in this book.

Until 1971 in Britain the mentally severely subnormal child was considered *ineducable*. His training was the responsibility of the Health Authorities and in the past had been considered to be occupational in nature. It is now felt that *all* children are educable in the true sense of the word. The mentally retarded child can be taught to function acceptably in many fields essential to normal living and some can be taught skills which will make them useful in adult life. Since April 1971 in Britain, these children's training has been the responsibility of the Education Authorities.

However, as a general rule it remains a fact that children with an IQ under 50 differ from those with IQs over 50 in several fairly clear ways.

a   Children with IQ under 50 usually show some evidence, either in the history or on clinical or psychological examination, of some form of brain pathology.

b   Because severe mental subnormality is usually due to brain pathology, it is likely that the child will have other physical defects.

c   Children with IQ under 50 achieve little success in learning the three Rs. Reading and writing at a simple level may be achieved. They are rarely able to do simple arithmetic.

d   As adults they are unlikely to be able to live independent lives and will have to live under sheltered conditions.

AETIOLOGY OF
MENTAL RETARDATION

The clinical conditions which give rise to brain pathology profound enough to depress the intelligence to a level where a normal independent life is impossible are numerous and ill-defined.

Socio-cultural

By the law of averages there will be a few mentally retarded children who show no organic cause for their low intelligence. The number of these children will balance that of those with superior intelligence of IQ 150 and upwards on the Gausserian curve. These mentally retarded children are born to parents of educationally subnormal level of intelligence, and are more intellectually disabled than their parents. The mental retardation is enhanced by poor living conditions and lack of opportunities for mental stimulation, such as encouragement to play, to explore and to listen to clear speech. Often these retarded children miss a considerable amount of school time, and leave school unable to read, poor in arithmetic and not yet able to hold down a job. They may be called social retardates. As there is no fundamental brain damage, this group is the most rewarding to train and educate. In a stimulating environment the IQ in this group may make a fairly quick apparent rise to 70 or more. These children will go on learning after leaving school. They will need help from the social services for many years. This is the group of mental retardates that may become delinquent. The girls may become promiscuous. There are a few of these children in training schools for the severely mentally subnormal. It is felt that usually they should not be placed with other retarded children such as those with Down's syndrome. They should have help in special classes in schools for the educationally subnormal. This type of child will later be capable of earning his living and marrying. The training he receives should have this end in view. Often in schools for the severely subnormal an odd child of this type shines as the pupil who is particularly good at performance skills but very poor on language development. This type of socially deprived, poorly endowed child is in a minority among a group of children with IQs under 50.

Malnutrition

It is possible that early malnutrition is a factor in the low intelligence of some socially deprived children and of some children from developing impoverished countries. It has been shown by Dobbing & Sands (1970) that the basic growth of the brain, as measured by the number of neutrons, continues up to 18 months of age. If a child suffers from malnutrition, and in particular protein lack, in the early years it may have a permanent adverse effect on intellectual potential. It is likely that children who suffered from kwashiorkor will be mentally retarded. Minor degrees of protein deprivation in early years may be a factor in the small heads, poor development and low intelligence of some children from deprived areas.

Genetic

Inherited conditions may account for about 5% of clearly defined disease entities and 3% of other cases of severe retardation where a specific diagnosis cannot be made.

Dominant Inheritance

These are few in number, as severely retarded people are unlikely to procreate and pass on a dominant gene. The term *phakomatosis* includes four conditions all associated with mental retardation: tuberous sclerosis, Sturge–Weber syndrome, the neuroretinal angiomatosis of Hippel–Landau type, and neurofibromatosis. The first condition is the commonest.

Tuberous Sclerosis   Children with this condition are mildly or severely retarded. There may be an early history of hypsarrhythmia, and many are epileptic. Adenoma sebaceum, an acneiform papular rash, appears on the face around the nose about the age of 5 years, and confirms the diagnosis. There are multiple potato-like nodules scattered irregularly through the nervous system and other parts of the body, often the heart and kidney. There may also be nodules on the skin and under the nails, and white naevi on the skin. A parent may have skin nodules or white naevi, confirming the dominant inheritance. After a few years intracerebral calcification can be seen by X-ray. There may be a sudden death. The condition may be a new mutation (Bundey 1970) in some families.

Sturge–Weber Syndrome   The child has a prominent naevus on one side of the face. There may be an angiomatous involvement of the choroid of the same side which can lead to glaucoma. There is an angiomatous involvement of the cortex and intracranial calcification is seen radiologically. There is usually a hemiparesis on the opposite side to the naevus. The majority of children are epileptic and mentally retarded.

Neurofibromatosis or von Recklinghausen's Disease   There are café-au-lait spots on the skin and neurofibromata distributed along the course of nerve roots, which may cause gigantism in a limb. Other skin lesions such as pigmented naevi, hypertrichosis or haemangiomata may be present. Children who have similar intracranial lesions are mentally retarded.

Recessive Inheritance

In these conditions both parents carry the same recessive gene which is passed on to an average of 1 in 4 of their children, explained in the following formula:

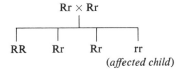

where R is the dominant gene and r the recessive gene carrying a pathological condition.

In mental retardation, many of the recessive genetic causes are biochemical in nature and some due to the failure of development of an essential enzyme in the metabolic chain of essential proteins or carbohydrates. The list of commoner known conditions to date of this type are given below and briefly described.

Phenylketonuria is the commonest type of biochemical defect. It occurs in 1 in 10,000 live births. The inborn enzyme defect is an inability to oxidise phenylalanine to tyrosine, and as a result phenylalanine accumulates in the blood and excess phenylpyruvic acid is excreted in the urine.

Phenylalanine in the blood can be detected after the baby has had 6 days of milk feeds by the Guthrie (1965) bacterial inhibition test. Unless the child is adequately treated, phenylpyruvic acid is present in the urine throughout life, and can be tested for in the clinic situation. A specimen of urine is acidified and a few drops of ferric chloride added. A greengage colour indicates the presence of phenylketonuria. A Phenostix reagent strip can be used.

A typical untreated case of this condition is severely mentally retarded. He always has fair to light brown hair and blue eyes. The reaching of all milestones is very delayed, but the children usually walk and learn to feed themselves. Speech is markedly delayed and may never appear. The children may develop bizarre mannerisms. They tend to twiddle their fingers and objects and pieces of string endlessly. The author has seen fourteen of this group all twiddling together—not copying one another—so it must be considered a definite organic sign. A fair number are epileptic. They often suffer from eczema. They can be difficult to handle, with tantrums and attacks of aggressiveness. There are wide variations in the degree of mental retardation, and some of the cases are later able to do simple factory work.

Affected children should be treated early on a low phenylalanine diet. The child is given a synthetic milk feed mixture, at first by bottle. Cereals, fruit and vegetables are allowed. Minimal amounts of phenylalanine must be present. On too strict a diet these children will not thrive, and death can occur. Some relaxation in the diet is possible in later childhood.

In expert hands, and with cooperation from parents and children, the outcome of dietary restriction can be good. It has been shown that, on the average, the earlier a phenylalanine low diet is instituted, the higher the eventual intelligence of the child.

Other but rarer types of mental retardation due to enzyme defects are briefly described:

Argininaemia and Argininosuccinicaciduria
Children have fine hair, hypotonia and a liability to vomit in early life. They may be epileptic.

Aspartyl Glucosaminuria
A number of cases have been reported from Finland. The children are short, with thickened skull and curved long bones. They have a broad nose, thickened lips and a large mouth.

Cystathioninuria and Homocystinuria
These two conditions are allied. Children with homocystinuria look very similar. They have fine fair hair and a marked malar flush. The legs are long and thin with genu valgum. The back shows kyphoscoliosis. Dislocation of the lens frequently occurs during childhood, and is accompanied by tremor of the iris. The children are liable to die of thrombosis. The abnormal amino acid in the urine is readily detected by a nitroprusside test. The condition can be ameliorated by a diet started early in life.

Galactosaemia
Due to an enzyme defect, there is a raised galactose level in the blood. Symptoms develop in the first few days of life. The baby is severely jaundiced and fails to thrive. Cataracts are present and frequently deafness. The liver is enlarged. Early cataracts in other members of the family may be an indication of dominant inheritance. The child must be reared on a lactose free diet.

Hartnup Disease
The children have an eczematous rash, brittle hair and intermittent cerebellar ataxia.

Histidinaemia
Children with this condition have a specific language disorder and the speech delay is out of proportion to the mental retardation. The urine gives a green colour with ferric chloride, similar to phenylketonuria. A diet has improved the condition. Some affected children may have normal intelligence, whilst their siblings are severely retarded.

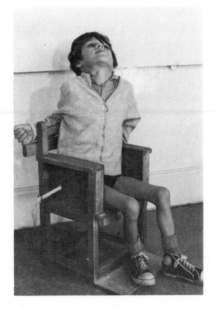

Fig. 11.1   A boy with ketotic hyperglycaemia, presenting as athetosis.

Hyperammonaemia
These mentally retarded children have episodes of severe vomiting from birth. The vision gradually deteriorates.

Hyperglycaemia
Ketotic and non-ketotic types. In the ketotic type the children have attacks of apnoea due to an upset in CO_2 metabolism. One child closely resembled an athetoid child (figure 11.1). Children with the non-ketotic variety may be only mildly retarded and attend a school for the educationally subnormal.

Hyperprolinaemia
This condition is associated with mild mental retardation and epilepsy.

Hyperuricaemia
Children, usually males, with this condition are easily recognised. They are hypotonic as babies and early in life develop choreiform movements, with an athetoid dance on attempting to walk. These children bite away their lips and fingers and appear to have a lack of sensation. Teeth may have

to be removed and the elbow joints restrained so that they cannot get their hands to their mouths. Speech may be present. There is an increased blood uric acid level (normal level 5 mg/100 ml). Uric acid crystals may occur in the urine.

Lowe's Syndrome (Cerebro-oculorenal syndrome)
These children have cataracts and are partially sighted, and they show marked hypotonia. There is proteinuria and aminoaciduria. The child has a vitamin-resistant rickets due to an inability of the renal tubules to reabsorb phosphate, and to balance this a loss of calcium from the bones. The bony deformities lead to an inability to walk in adolescence. Large doses of vitamin D may ameliorate the condition.

Maple Syrup Disease
The children are epileptic, often show rigidity and have eczema. There is a peculiar smell to the urine. The diagnosis is made in infancy by a positive dinitrophenylhydrazine test.

Refsum's Syndrome
There are abnormalities of fatty acid metabolism. The children are profoundly retarded, blind due to retinitis, and show evidence of polyneuritis and cerebellar ataxia. The condition may be allied to a lipoidosis.

All these conditions are seen from time to time in any clinical paediatric practice. The diagnosis should be made early, as many are amenable to dietary treatment.

Diagnosis and supervision of treatment require the services of an expert biochemist and a dietician. It may be preferable to transfer a child to a hospital whose staff have a particular interest in the condition. Long-distance supervision may be possible with outpatient and inpatient assessments at intervals.

Other Metabolic Disorders

Hypercalcaemia

The baby is markedly hypotonic at birth, and causes concern by frequent vomiting, constipation and polyuria. A raised serum calcium as high as 36 mg/100 ml has been recorded in a 7-week breast-fed baby. The child develops into a dwarf with epilepsy and a typical elfin face. There may be atherosclerosis. Calcium is deposited in the kidneys, and may be the eventual cause of death. Cardiac defects such as aortic stenosis may be present. The condition should be diagnosed early, as it will respond to a reduced intake of calcium and vitamin D.

Lipid and Mucopolysaccharide Disorders

Children with these conditions show progressive neurological deterioration, due to neuronal storage of abnormal material, either lipids or mucopolysaccharides.

Gargoylism These children are stunted in growth, and have an abnormal body configuration (figure 11.2). Various types, with different genetic inheritance and intellectual deficit, are shown in table 11.1.

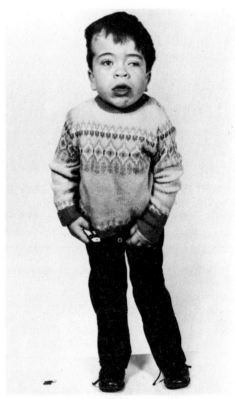

Fig. 11.2 Hurler's syndrome

Table 11.1 Mucopolysaccharide Disorders

Type	Clinical Condition	Abnormalities in Urine and Marrow

Hurler	Autosomal recessive
	Mentally retarded
	Stunted
	Thoracic deformities
	Flat nasal bridge
	Thick lips and tongue
	Broad tip to nose
	Wide nostrils
	Open mouth
	Liver and spleen enlarged
	Stiff joints
	X-ray Wedge vertebrae
	            with anterior beaking
	        Short phalanges
	        Corneal clouding
	        Cardiovascular
	            complications
		Chondroitin sulphate B
		Heparitin sulphate

Hunter	Clinically similar to Hurler Sex-linked recessive Deafness may occur No corneal clouding No CVS complications	Chondroitin sulphate B Heparitin sulphate
Sanfilippo	Autosomal recessive Deafness Retinitis pigmentosa No corneal clouding No stunting No CVS lesions *X-ray* Thick skull vault	Heparitin sulphate
Morquio	Autosomal recessive Mentally fairly normal Skeletal changes	Kerato sulphate
Scheie	Autosomal recessive Mentally normal Hairy Not stunted Stiff joints Aortic valve disease	Chondroitin sulphate B

Amaurotic Family Idiocy (Tay-Sachs, Bielschowsky, Spielmayer Vogt, Ku's diseases) An apparently normal child begins to deteriorate between the ages of 4 and 6 months. There is hypotonia, myoclonic epilepsy and rapid onset of blindness. A diagnostic sign is a cherry red spot at the macula and retinal changes. Death occurs by 2 years. It is commoner in the Jewish race.

Niemann-Pick Disease The condition commences in early life and is biochemically similar to Tay-Sachs disease. There is no cherry red spot at the macula. The liver, spleen and sometimes lymph glands become enlarged.

Gaucher's Disease The condition begins in childhood. There is mental deterioration with enlargement of liver and spleen. Typical Gaucher cells are found in the spleen and lymph glands. There is a raised acid phosphatase.

Leucodystrophies

There is degeneration of the myelin in the white matter of the cerebrum and the peripheral nerves, and in consequence the child shows progressive dementia, blindness, epilepsy and cerebral palsy. Several types are described: Krabbe's disease, Merzbacher-Pelizaeus disease and metachromatic leucodystrophy. In metachromatic leucodystrophy, abnormal breakdown products can be detected in the urine.

These conditions are autosomal recessive in nature. It is important to make a diagnosis, as the chance of further affected children is 1 : 4. The diagnosis may be made by examination of a small portion of cerebral cortex after cerebral biopsy, or of the nerve fibres in a resected layer of the rectum. It has been found safer and more satisfactory to remove the appendix for full examination of the nerve fibres by a neuropathologist. The operation causes little upset to a severely retarded child.

Deteriorating conditions are seen fairly frequently in hospitals for the subnormal; and the diagnosis, if made, must be conveyed to parents. The differential diagnosis is a subacute encephalitis, possibly following measles, which is not of genetic significance.

Other Recessive Conditions

Microcephaly   A small head, noticeable at birth, with no evidence of antenatal or perinatal brain damage, may be a recessive condition. A guarded opinion must be given about the possibility of other affected children. Often these children are generally rigid and give a superficial appearance of spasticity. The rigidity appears to be due to a cocontraction of agonists and antagonists, and can be reduced with early movement training. These microcephalic children can grow up to be adults with useful skills and abilities. They can learn domestic tasks.

Spastic Quadriplegia   A child may have an entirely normal birth and later show evidence of severe spasticity and mental retardation and epilepsy. The condition can be recessively inherited. The author has known seven cases where a later sibling was similarly affected. This emphasises the fact that where there is no evidence of perinatal pathology the condition may be one of recessive inheritance. The difficulty arises when the child has a difficult birth with neonatal problems and the spastic quadriplegia is later proved by the birth of a similarly affected child to be one of recessive inheritance. The abnormal birth was fortuitous. These cases emphasise the need to be guarded in all genetic advice.

Chromosome Anomalies

Conditions due to abnormal mitosis at the time of conception—which are usually associated with mental retardation—are briefly described.

Down's Syndrome (Mongolism)

The incidence is about 1 in every 600 births and occurs throughout the world from Greenland to Japan. Children with Down's syndrome are more likely to be born to older mothers; the incidence where the mother is aged 40 years or over is 1 in 45. These children have 47 chromosomes instead of the usual 46, and the extra chromosome is in the 21/22 group—trisomy 21/22.

Translocation   3% of mongols have only 46 chromosomes. There has been a translocation of part of one chromosome to the 21/22 group. The mother is likely to have 45 chromosomes, with a translocation of the missing chromosome on to another group. She is likely to give birth to further mongol children.

Mosaicism A child with the typical appearance of mongolism may have only a proportion of cells with 47 chromosomes, a phenomenon called mosaicism. These children are not necessarily more intelligent than other mongols.

The condition can be diagnosed at birth. The child has the typical upward slant of eyes, epicanthic folds, Brushfield's spots in the irides, primitive ears, flat occiput and low placed thumbs. A constant factor is a fissured tongue. They are always hypotonic as babies, with poor head control for several months. If there is any doubt about the diagnosis, chromosome examination should be done immediately. Mongols often have other congenital abnormalities. A cardiac septal defect occurs in 8–10%. The child may have cataracts, cleft palate, diaphragmatic hernia or imperforate anus. It is not generally realised that a fair proportion are deaf.

Later on the child with Down's syndrome is more liable to have nasal catarrh, bronchitis and diarrhoea. A few—more than generally recorded—are epileptic. Cataracts may develop in adolescence and should be specifically looked for at intervals.

The majority of these children grow up to be happy, pleasant children with an IQ around 30–40. They may show a streak of obstinacy. They appear very unaffected by their environment and will remain placid and happy when the world around them is in chaos. Nearly all of them achieve walking, slightly later than normal. They talk late and are often disappointingly indistinct and monosyllabic. Toilet training and skill in feeding themselves are usually achieved. They can take part in an active training situation. They may learn to dance, sew and cook, and later do simple factory work.

There are a few disappointing cases of profound subnormality where independent walking and self-help are never achieved. A few, on the other hand, do better than expected, and learn to read and do very simple arithmetic. Occasionally, usually in rural areas, a mongol achieves independent employment.

These children live longer now than they did thirty years ago, due to the use of antibiotics. There is still an increased mortality rate throughout childhood and adolescence, so that only a few reach 40 to 50 years of age.

Cri-du-Chat Syndrome

This condition is due to partial deletion of the short arm of chromosome 5. In a certain percentage of cases, one parent has an abnormal chromosome pattern, so chromosome examination of the parents should be made. These children are noted to have a cat-mew cry as babies. They are profoundly subnormal and late in walking. There is a high early death rate.

Patau's Syndrome

This condition is due to an extra chromosome in the 13/15 group—trisomy 13/15. The child is severely retarded and has multiple congenital abnormalities, such as a cardiac defect, cleft lip and palate, polydactyly and ear deformities. He dies early.

Edward's Syndrome

In this condition there is trisomy 17/18. The patients are short in stature, with hypertonicity, multiple congenital abnormalities and typical rocker bottom feet.

Abnormality of Sex Chromosome

Children with Turner's syndrome (XO abnormality), Klinefelter's syndrome (XXY abnormality) or various XXX or XXXY or XYY abnormalities are found among a population of mentally subnormal cases. The clinical condition may vary from profound retardation, educational subnormality, to symptoms suggestive of autism or gross aggressiveness.

It is thought that all mentally retarded children with abnormal facies, epicanthic folds, low placed ears, broad hands, abnormal palm prints or multiple congenital abnormalities should have a chromosome examination. Abnormal findings, such as an abnormally long arm of the Y chromosome or an extra ring chromosome, may be found. The significance of some of these findings is not yet clear.

Syndromes which include Mental Retardation

There are a number of syndromes associated with mental retardation for which a biochemical or cytogenetic cause has not yet been found. The number of these syndromes increases annually as more children with similar characteristics are described. Pictures or atlases of these conditions may help with the diagnosis. The more common are described below.

Apert's Syndrome (acrocephalosyndactyly) The child's skull is high and shortened anteroposteriorly. The eyes are prominent and widely set, with an antimongoloid slant. The palate is high and sometimes cleft. There are anomalies of the hands and fingers, with fusion of digits.

Cockayne's Syndrome These children are dwarfs with long limbs and eye abnormalities—retinal degeneration, optic atrophy or cataracts. They show early senility (progeria).

Crouzon's Disease Craniostenosis causes an abnormally shaped head, hypoplasia of the maxilla, prognathism, exophthalmos and a beaked nose. The condition may be alleviated if the craniostenosis is noted early.

De Lange Syndrome (Amsterdam dwarf) The child has a brachycephalic skull, confluent eyebrows, upturned nose, long upper lip, general hairiness and frequent severe abnormalities of the arm, hands and feet. There may be an abnormal ring chromosome.

Ehlers–Danlos Syndrome The child has hyperelastic skin and overabundance of connective tissue and hyperextensive joints. There are frequent haemorrhages, epilepsy and club feet.

Franceschetti's (oculoauriculovertebral dysplasia: Goldenhar's syndrome) Congenital abnormalities include dermoids, colobomata, microphthalmia, microtia, micrognathus, verebral anomalies and congenital heart disease.

Hallerman–Streiff Syndrome The children are dwarfs with beaked noses, small mouths, microphthalmos, cataracts and sparse hair on the head. The intelligence may be surprisingly high.

Hallevorden–Spatz Syndrome This diagnosis is made at post mortem in a mentally defective patient who has slowly deteriorated and shown progressive rigidity, athetosis and epilepsy. There is a rusty brown discolouration of the basal ganglia.

Happy Puppet Syndrome   The child has a small head with a flat occiput, protruding tongue and hypotonia. Infantile spasms occur. The child is easily provoked to senseless laughter.

Kinky Hair Syndrome (Memke's syndrome)   The child has a small head with micrognathos and a high arched palate. The scalp hair is sparse and kinky. There is rapid neurological deterioration and the child dies in infancy.

Klipper–Feil Syndrome   These children have a short neck due to synostosis of the cervical vertebrae. The head appears to arise directly from the chest. There may be cerebellar ataxia and epilepsy.

Laurence–Moon–Biedl Syndrome   The child shows polydactylism (six fingers and toes), hypogenitalism, retinal pigmentation with defective vision and obesity.

Leprechaunism   The child is of short stature, with hirsutism and an emaciated 'old man' face. There are various endocrine abnormalities. Death occurs early.

Pendred's Syndrome   The child is deaf, with an enlarged thyroid gland. This condition is usually euthyroid.

Pierre Robin Syndrome   These children have micrognathus, cleft palate and harelip, and are generally small and retarded, with bird-like faces. Feeding is difficult in infancy.

Prader–Willi Syndrome   At birth the child is markedly hypotonic. There may be feeding difficulties. Later in childhood he becomes extremely obese. The genitalia remain infantile. Diabetes is likely to occur in adolescence.

Rubinstein–Taybi Syndrome   The patient has a broad forehead and long upper lip; but the distinctive feature of the condition is broad and often duplicated thumbs and big toes.

Sjögren–Larsson Syndrome   This condition has been extensively investigated in England by Richards (1970). There is ichthyosis, spasticity of a diplegic type and mental retardation. There may be epilepsy.

Smith–Lemli–Opitz Syndrome   The head is long and there is a broad bridge of nose with upturned nares and increased nasolabial folds. There may be hypospadias and skeletal abnormalities. The child vomits frequently as a baby, and pyloric stenosis is common.

Soto's Syndrome (cerebral gigantism)   The child is large in weight and height from birth. The skull is doliocephalic with prognathism and an antimongoloid slant to the eyes. There is enlargement of the cerebral ventricles.

Treacher Collins' Syndrome   These patients are quite distinctive and can be diagnosed at a distance. They have prominent bat-ears with primitive pattern, an underdeveloped maxilla, giving hollow cheeks, and an antimongoloid slant to the eyes. There is usually an extremely high palate and crowded teeth, with an associated speech defect. It is thought to be due to a failure of development of the first vertebral arch and may be associated with deafness. Mental retardation may not be a feature.

Virchow–Seckel Syndrome   The baby is born light for dates and has a bird-like appearance. The child later is dwarfed in size, has a small head, hypoplasia of the malar bones, a prominent beaked nose, a high arched palate and micrognathos. There may be joint dislocations.

Abnormalities of Skull and Brain

Many congenital abnormalities of the central nervous system, whether due to genetic, cytogenetic or developmental influences, will be secondarily responsible for mental retardation.

Microcephaly is common among mentally subnormal individuals. The head circumference is at least three standard deviations less than the mean. There is a genetic form of the condition. It may occur in many of the syndromes mentioned. Diseases in pregnancy, such as toxoplasmosis or rubella, malnutrition or placental insufficiency, may cause delayed development. The growth of the skull may be retarded postnatally, due to perinatal or postnatal damage to the brain. The absence of growth of soft tissue may prevent bony growth. The condition may be due to abnormally early closure of the sutures, as in craniostenosis. This condition can be suspected when the skull circumference in infancy ceases to increase, and a ridge of bony overgrowth can be felt along the suture line, the coronal and/or saggital sutures. Early surgery to open up the sutures can prevent mental retardation if the condition is noted early.

Hydrocephaly   In these children the head circumference is more than three standard deviations greater than normal and there may be evidence that the head circumference is increasing unduly rapidly. The condition may be due to a blockage in the flow of cerebrospinal fluid, such as an aqueduct stenosis, or an acquired blockage due to meningitis or the Arnold–Chiari abnormality in myelomeningocele. The child typically has a bulging fontanelle, a prominent forehead and sunset eyes. Surgery for the insertion of a shunt mechanism may be performed; but the eventual outcome for the child may not be perfect. Epilepsy, defective sight, low intelligence and learning problems may follow.

Hydranencephaly is a congenital defect in which large areas of the cortex are replaced by a membranous sac containing cerebrospinal fluid, and is a more severe form of porencephaly.

Abnormal Shaped Skulls   Mentally retarded children frequently have abnormally shaped skulls. The underlying brain may have a developmental defect.

Brachycephaly is the term used for an unusually round head with a flattened occipital region. It may occur after birth injury involving the occipital lobe, and may be associated with cerebral blindness.

Scaphocephaly describes an excessively long head in the antero-posterior direction. It may be due to early closure of the sagittal suture.

Plagiocephaly describes a markedly asymmetrical head.

Acrocephaly (turricephaly) describes a tall head, shortened antero-posteriorly, and is seen in Apert's syndrome.

Hyperostosis is a condition where bone is deposited on the inner aspect of the frontal bones, causing lack of brain development.

Cranium Bifida   Associated with the abnormal head shape there may be anomalies such as encephalocele. This may occur anteriorly between the eyes or posteriorly in the occipital region.

Associated with the skull abnormality there may be an abnormal slant to eyes, abnormally shaped or low placed ears, hypertelorism, defective maxillary development of face (as in Treacher Collins' syndrome) or micrognathos (as in Pierre Robin syndrome). An abnormal looking head and face are frequently associated with mental retardation, but this is not invariably the case. Turricephaly, Treacher Collins' syndrome and other skull abnormalities are seen in adult patients with normal intelligence.

Endocrine Disorders

Hypothyroidism (Cretinism)

This is the commonest endocrine cause of mental retardation; and even this condition is not as common as originally thought, when the word cretin was synonymous with mental retardation. It occurs in about 1 case in 600 of mental retardation. The absence of the thyroid gland may be developmental or due to absence of iodine in the mother's diet. The child develops normally for a few weeks and then becomes pale, puffy and anaemic. He may develop a greenish hue. There is a large tongue, supraclavicular pads of fat and an umbilical hernia, with delayed bone age, low serum protein-bound iodine level and raised blood cholesterol. The child grows up to be a thick-set dwarf of very small stature, unless he is adequately treated from birth with thyroid or one of the extracts of the thyroid gland. An affected adult is rarely seen today, due to early treatment.

Diabetes Insipidus

There is an inability to concentrate urine due to a deficiency of the posterior pituitary hormone, vasopressin. Severe polyuria may cause mental retardation due to dehydration and hypernatraemia in the first weeks of life. With adequate early treatment and maintenance of a normal electrolyte balance, mental retardation need not occur. The condition is transmitted as a sex-linked recessive.

Antenatal Causes of Mental Retardation

Maternal Infections Leading to Mental Retardation

Rubella is responsible for the condition in some deaf-blind children.

Toxoplasmosis causes microcephaly or hydrocephaly and microphthalmia.

Syphilis, because of antenatal supervision and treatment, is a rare cause nowadays.

Influenza has been considered a possible teratogenic agent.

Cytomegalic Inclusion Body Disease causes similar effects to toxoplasmosis. There may be intracerebral calcification.

Smoking

Butler (1972) has shown that smoking in pregnancy is directly related to lowered intelligence in the child. Whether excessive smoking in pregnancy can cause severe mental subnormality is not yet established.

Irradiation

Irradiation to the pelvic organs in the early weeks of pregnancy has been known to cause damage to the developing fetal central nervous system. The child is in danger of microcephaly and mental retardation.

Drugs

The thalidomide disaster has highlighted the damage to the fetus of the maternal intake of drugs in early pregnancy; and numerous so-called cytotoxic drugs have been blamed. Quinine, certain antibiotics and salicylates have been named. Mental retardation in the baby may follow carbon monoxide poisoni   during pregnancy.

Perinatal Causes

In the conditions already described, mental retardation has been related to abnormal development before birth. In many cases the child looks abnormal. The fact that development was abnormal from early pregnancy is confirmed if the palm and finger prints are abnormal. Abnormalities of this type are seen particularly in children with an abnormal chromosome karyotype. There are a considerable number of mentally retarded children who show no congenital abnormalities, and where the evidence suggests that the brain pathology has been caused at the time of birth. Assessing the child population in a hospital for the subnormal, the author felt that in about 10% of the children brain pathology at the time of birth could be considered the likely cause.

There may be a history of maternal toxaemia followed by neonatal asphyxia in the baby. The baby may have been markedly premature by dates and have given cause for concern soon after birth. Other babies may have been born after a 40-week gestation period, but have been light for dates, i.e. under 2500 grams birth weight. Light for dates babies are 'at risk' of becoming hypoglycaemic soon after birth. Brain damage from hypoglycaemia can be prevented by early high calorie feeding. Other retarded children have been born after a prolonged labour followed by a forceps, breech or Caesarian birth, and subsequent neonatal complications. There is a higher than normal incidence of twin births among retardates. In one ward of 50 mentally subnormal women, of whom a number were spastics, 8 were twins. There is a frequent history of postmaturity, which may be significant if, in addition, there has been an antepartum haemorrhage which may have caused placental separation and later insufficiency. After birth neonatal jaundice may give rise to brain damage leading to athetosis and deafness. It has been found that convulsions in the first three days of life and after the eighth day are likely to be followed by mental retardation. Neonatal convulsions in the third to eighth day only may be due to hypocalcaemia, which carries a less serious prognosis.

Postnatal Causes

Illnesses during infancy and childhood can lead to mental retardation. These include all forms of meningitis and encephalitis. Encephalitis following measles is particularly liable to leave a child epileptic and spastic. There is often a bilateral hemiplegia and retardation. Convulsions and permanent brain damage are unfortunate rare sequelae of immunisations. Lead poisoning from chewing paint or putty with a high lead content may lead to a gradual deterioration, resembling autism with permanent brain damage and epilepsy. Asphyxia under anaesthesia or from near drowning or cardiac arrest may lead to permanent brain damage. Cerebral malaria has caused mental retardation in children from mosquito infested countries. Cerebrovascular anomalies, thromboses and cerebral tumours may cause cerebral palsy and retardation. Accidents, either on the road or following the battered baby syndrome, may leave permanent brain damage. These last two causes are becoming commoner.

Cases with No Known Aetiology

There remain a high proportion of cases—the percentage varies widely in different surveys—where no exact aetiology can be attached to the condition. The child may be born to a healthy, happily married couple with no adverse genetic family history after a planned pregnancy. The birth may have been entirely normal and there has been no concern in the neonatal period. Yet the child is found later to be severely subnormal. There may be no minor congenital abnormalities to suggest a developmental cause. One presumes that conditions such as anoxia, hypoglycaemia or placental insufficiency may have been undetected at birth. There may have been an ill-defined virus encephalitis. In some cases there may be brain anomalies undetected during life, such as a defect of the corpus callosum. The birth of a similarly affected sibling may reveal an autosomal recessive causation. In some cases there is no abnormality to be detected at post mortem.

ADDITIONAL HANDICAPS

With this wide range of clinical conditions likely to produce mental retardation, it is not surprising that the child frequently has other physical handicaps. A mentally retarded child is a multiple handicapped child.

Visual Defects

There is an above average incidence of refractive errors. Myopia is particularly common in children with Down's syndrome and also following a premature birth. Hypermetropia may occur in children with cerebral palsy. Eye movement defects—nystagmus, strabismus and cranial nerve abnormalities—are very common. There may be an undetected field of vision defect or tunnel vision. Lens, media, retinal and optic nerve defects may be present. Many children may show evidence of cerebral blindness.

Because it is often difficult to make sure how much a mentally retarded child can see, a full refraction should take place on *every* child. His eyes should be examined by an ophthalmologist, under an anaesthetic if necessary.

Hearing Defects

It should be a firm rule that all children with mental retardation are tested by an audiologist using all modern facilities. Methods such as distraction techniques and free-field audiometry may give a satisfactory result. With these children evoked response audiometry may be employed, although the result obtained may not be more satisfactory than good clinical observation. Hearing aids should not be given to a mentally retarded child unless the hearing loss has been fully confirmed, as this may delay the child's learning of auditory discrimination.

Epilepsy

All the conditions listed above may be associated with epilepsy. There may be an occasional seizure or more frequent fits occurring several times a day. The epilepsy may take many forms, and bizarre types of epilepsy are found in hospitals for the subnormal. An EEG should, if possible, be a routine investigation, and the recording should be analysed by an expert who may be able to advise on medication. The medication for each case must be supervised very closely. It is not unusual to find a child or adult who has unfortunately continued to take medication when there have been no fits for years. It is also possible to find children who are having exactly the same type and number of fits after a prolonged period of medication. Deterioration on drugs may not be spotted, unless reports are regularly received from parents and teachers. There is a particular danger with phenytoin medication. The child or adolescent may have become ataxic and flexed, even to the extent of no longer being able to walk, after a period on epanutin medication. At the same time, the convulsions may not have been controlled. In these cases, there is a low serum folate level and reduced mineral content of bone. Possibly all patients on prolonged epanutin medication should have routine serum folate investigations; and with levels below 4 mg/ml the medication should be changed. Routine neurological examinations are necessary with all children on anticonvulsants.

In a hospital for subnormals, it has been found that as many as 30% are epileptics receiving medication.

Movement Defects

All types of movement defects are common in mental retardation. Apart from the typical cases of hemiplegia, bilateral hemiplegia, spastic diplegia and athetosis, there are children with odd incoordinated movements. Some have tremors and abnormally delayed balance reactions. In some the delayed mobility appears to be related to a severe body image defect and a lack of orientation of themselves in space. Movement defects should be analysed so that appropriate help can be given. Muscular dystrophy, Friedreich's ataxia and dystrophia myotonica may develop during childhood in mentally retarded children. Increased motor incoordination may be the early signs of a deteriorating neurological condition.

Speech Defects

Speech defects and communication disorders are common. Apart from the mental retardation, the child may have a dysarthria or dyspraxia. The abilities in receptive and expressive language may be below what might be expected from the performance skills.

BEHAVIOUR DISORDERS

There are some behaviour disorders among retarded children which are specifically related to the brain pathology. These include hyperactivity, lack of concentration and distractibility. There is evidence that aggressiveness may be due to an XYY chromosome abnormality or to a temporal lobe defect. Autism or autistic features in a mental retardate are likely to be due to brain pathology and the inability of the child to translate the clues he is receiving from sensory stimuli.

It is felt that many of these difficulties are created by the abnormal environment in which the child lives, and are only secondarily related to the brain damage. Some children have been rejected by their parents from birth. Admission to a hospital for the subnormal in very early childhood may cause a severe emotional disturbance. These children may never develop a sense of their own identity. They may never have known a mother figure or had personal possessions. They may show severe disturbances, such as aggressiveness, self destruction and withdrawal.

Alternatively, the demands to conform in a home environment may be too exacting for the child; and he may react by hyperactive and destructive behaviour. These children may improve in behaviour if removed to a less demanding but home-like hostel.

There are undoubtedly some severely mentally retarded children who show antisocial and unacceptable behaviour as part of the pattern of low intelligence.

Staff dealing with mentally retarded people—children and adults—have to be specifically trained to cope with behaviour problems, because they are so frequent and difficult to handle. They can include very offensive behaviour, such as biting themselves and others, playing with saliva and smearing faeces. Homosexual behaviour and open masturbation become problems to the staff handling groups of adolescent mental retardates.

The behaviour of mentally retarded children can however usually be considered as a reaction to their environment, and the difficult behaviour can be seen as a reaction to conditions imposed on the child by reason of his handicap, either as frustration of natural desires, or intolerance of institutional standards, routine or unenlightened treatment.

REFERENCES

ALLEN J A & HOLT K S (1972) *Biochemical Approaches to Mental Handicap in Children.* Churchill, London

ANGELI E & KIRMAN B H (1970) Genetic counselling of the family of the mentally retarded child. *Proceedings of the 2nd Congress of the International Association for the Scientific Study of Mental Deficiency (Warsaw)*, 692

BENDA C E (1960) *The Child with Mongolism.* Grune & Stratton, New York

BERG J, MCCREARY B, RIDLER M A C & SMITH G F (1970) *The De Lange Syndrome.* Pergamon, Oxford

BICKEL H (1967) The treatment of phenylketonuria. In *Conferences on Phenylketonuria and Allied Disorders.* Children's Bureau, Washington 99

BITTER T, MUIR H, MITTWOCH U & SCOTT J D (1966) A contribution to the differential diagnosis of Hurler's disease and forms of Morguior syndrome. *J. Bone Jt. Surg.* **48**, 4

BRENTON D P (1969) Treatment of homocystinuria. *Dev. Med. Childh. Neurol.* **11**, 4, 59

BUNDEY S (1970) Genetic counselling in relation to tuberous sclerosis. *Dev. Med. Childh. Neurol*, 699

BUTLER N R & BONHAM D G (1963) *Perinatal Mortality.* Livingstone, Edinburgh

CABABSKA B ET AL (1970) Evaluation of early treatment. *Proceedings of the 2nd Congress of the International Association for the Scientific Study of Mental Deficiency, Warsaw*, 253

CARTER C H (1965) *Medical Aspects of Mental Retardation.* C C Thomas, Springfield, Illinois

CARTER C H (1966) *Mental Retardation Syndromes.* C C Thomas, Springfield, Illinois

CROME L C & STERN J (1967) *The Pathology of Mental Retardation.* Churchill, London

DEPARTMENT OF HEALTH AND SOCIAL SECURITY (1972) *Human Genetics* Department of Health and Social Security, London

DOBBING J & SANDS J (1970) Undernutrition and the developing brain. *Proceedings of the 2nd Congress of the International Association for the Scientific Study of Mental Deficiency, Warsaw*, 476

FORD F R (1966) *Diseases of the Nervous System in Infancy, Childhood and Adolescence.* Blackwell, Oxford

GELLIS S S & FEINGOLD M (1968) *Atlas of Mental Retardation Syndromes.* U.S. Department of Health, Education and Welfare, Washington

GOODMAN J & TIZARD J (1962) Prevalence of imbecility and idiocy among children. *Brit. med. J.* **1**, 216

GORDON N (1970) Delayed speech and hirtidinaemia. *Dev. Med. Childh. Neurol.* **12**, 1, 104

GORDON N & THURSBY-PELHAM O (1969) The Sanfilippo syndrome. *Dev. Med. Childh. Neurol.* **11**, 4, 485

GORDON R R & LEJEUNE J (1965) The cri du chat syndrome. *Dev. Med. Childh. Neurol.* **55**, 453

GUTHRIE R & WHITNEY S (1965) *Phenylketonuria Detection in the Newborn Infant as a Routine Hospital Procedure.* U.S. Department of Health, Education and Welfare Administration, Washington

HAMERTON J ed. (1964) *Chromosomes in Medicine. Clinics in Developmental Medicine* No. 5 Spastics Society & William Heinemann, London

HILLIARD L T & KIRMAN B H (1965) *Mental Deficiency.* Churchill, London

HOLDER J D (1967) The Russell Silver dwarf. *Dev. Med. Childh. Neurol.* **9**, 4, 457

Hsia D Y Y (1970) Phenylketonuria, clinical, genetic and biochemical aspects. *Proceedings of the Congress of the 2nd International Association for the Scientific Study of Mental Deficiency, Warsaw,* 105

Kirman B H (1964) Cretinism. *Dev. Med. Childh. Neurol.* **6**, 3, 306

Kirman B H (1972) *The Mentally Handicapped Child.* Nelson, London

O'Connor N & Hermelin B (1963) *Speech and Thought in Severe Subnormality.* Pergamon, Oxford

Opitz J M (1969) Genetic malformation syndromes associated with mental retardation. *Congenital Mental Retardation,* pp. 209-225. University of Texas, Austin

Palo J et al (1970) Clinical characteristics of aspartylglucosaminuria. *Proceedings of the 2nd Congress of the International Association for the Scientific Study of Mental Deficiency, Warsaw*

Partingdon M W & Hennen B K E (1967) The Lesch Nylar syndrome. *Dev. Med. Childh. Neurol.* **9**, 5, 563

Patau K (1964) *Partial Trisomy. Conf. Cong. Malformations,* pp. 52-9. Int. Med. Congr. Ltd. New York

Paulson G W & Lyle C A (1966) Tuberous sclerosis. *Devel. Med. Childh. Neurol.* **5,** 571

Penrose L S (1938) *A Clinical and Genetic Study of 1280 Cases of Mental Defect.* MRC Special Report Series, No. 229. HMSO, London

Penrose L S (1963) *The Biology of Mental Defect.* Sidgwick & Jackson, London

Penrose L S & Smith G F (1966) *Down's Anomaly.* Churchill, London

Penrose L S (1970) Mental ability and chromosome errors. *Proceedings of the 2nd Congress of the International Association for the Scientific Study of Mental Deficiency, Warsaw,* 79

Proceedings of the First Congress of the International Association for the Scientific Study of Mental Deficiency, Montpelier (1967) Michael Jackson, London

Proceedings of the Second Congress of the International Association for the Scientific Study of Mental Deficiency, Warsaw (1970) Polish Medical Publishers, Warsaw

Richards B (1970) The Sjögren-Larsson syndrome. *Proceedings of the 2nd Congress of the International Association for the Scientific Study of Mental Deficiency, Warsaw,* 367

Rubinstein J H & Taybi H (1963) Broad thumbs and toes and facial abnormalities. *Amer. J. Dis. Child.* **105**, 588

Schwaite J F & Kolendrianos E T (1969) Maple syrup urine disease. *Dev. Med. Childh. Neurol.* **11**, 4, 460

Smithells R W (1965) De Lange's Amsterdam dwarf syndrome. *Dev. Med. Childh. Neurol.* **1**, 27

Stanbury J B, Wyngaarden J B & Fredrickson D S (1966) *The Metabolic Basis of Inherited Disease.* McGraw-Hill, New York

Taylor A L (1967) Patau Edwards cri du chat syndrome. *Dev. Med. Childh. Neurol.* **1**, 78

Westall R G (1963) Maple syrup urine disease. Dietary treatment. *Arch. Dis. Childh.* **38**, 485

Wilson J (1972) Investigation of degenerative disease of the central nervous system. *Arch. Dis. Childh.* **47**, 252, 163

Chapter 12
Management of the Mentally Retarded Child

PAEDIATRIC ADVICE

The paediatrician's first contact with a mentally retarded child may be in the neonatal period. This is particularly true with mongols, who can usually be diagnosed with confidence immediately after birth. At one time parents were not told that their child was abnormal until several months after birth, when they had already realised that he was not developing normally. There are some doctors who feel this delay is right. However the decision when to tell the parents has been taken out of the doctor's hands. With information from television and popular journals, members of the general population can recognise a mongol, and the parents are likely to be given the information in an unpredictable manner. The parents should be told of the child's condition as soon after the birth as the emotional state of the mother permits, either by a paediatrician or by a family doctor, with both parents present. The paediatrician can give a short explanation of the condition and answer questions. The parents should be given another early appointment for discussion. At a second interview they will have more questions to ask, and it may be found that they have serious misconceptions.

'At Risk' Register

Children with abnormally small heads or congenital abnormalities may be diagnosed at birth as potentially mentally retarded. If there has been a difficult or abnormal birth, or the child has been seriously ill in the neonatal period, it may be suspected from birth that he will not develop normally. The names of these children should be on an 'at risk' register, and they should be seen regularly by a paediatrician, a local authority doctor or a family doctor.

Delayed Development

There will be a number of children who, although born after a normal pregnancy and having a normal birth and neonatal period, develop abnormally and are later found to be mentally retarded. It is still not proved whether the abnormality could have been predicted by a neurological examination at 1 week of age. A health visitor, recording the milestones of all children in her district, is likely to be the first one after the parents to be alerted to possible retardation.

Investigation

A child who is not developing normally should be referred without delay to a paediatrician. It is justifiable to do a full work-up of clinical and pathological investigations in every case. After a history has been taken and a clinical examination has been made, the investigations should include:

1 X-ray of skull and wrist for bone age
2 Urine chromatography to exclude abnormal aminoaciduria
3 Examination of the urine for abnormal sugars
4 Estimation of serum calcium, phosphorus and alkaline phosphatase
5 Immunological assays for rubella, toxoplasmosis and cytomegalic viruses in the early months of life
6 Tests for syphilis
7 EEG examination
8 Where there are specific indications, chromosome analysis and estimations of protein-bound iodine, blood lead and uric acid levels may be carried out. If gargoylism is suspected a 24-hour specimen or urine should be examined for mucopolysaccharides.

Some clinicians have queried the value of all these investigations in every case. A clinician versed in mental subnormality can often make the diagnosis without them. There is always the argument that they may be of no help to the child. There are a considerable number of children in whom all investigations are negative. Over the years one has become increasingly convinced of the value of full investigations. Frequently there are odd cases where the investigations reveal the diagnosis: Turner's syndrome in a child, cri-du-chat syndrome, Lowe's syndrome. These may be of help when one is giving advice about the future, and in providing genetic advice. Experience with adults has also emphasised the need for full investigations. If the child's condition is not documented when young, he may later live as an adult in a residential home or hospital and nothing will be on record about the early history. When fits develop in adult life it may not be known that he had fits in infancy. Intracranial calcification may be noted in adult life, and there is nothing known about the patient to help with aetiology. I have known a woman of 60 years, crippled in adult life due to a spinal tumour, when it was wrongly assumed that she had had spastic diplegia from birth. Even the onset of cataracts and blindness may not be recorded. This confusion is frequently the experience of doctors looking after a group of adults, and emphasises the need for full documentation in childhood, when the parents are able to give a clear history. Regular follow-up records of progress should be kept.

Making a rare diagnosis on a child in this group of interesting medical conditions has been called 'stamp collecting', and may be of limited value. We should also be recording and investigating ways in which the mentally subnormal differ from the normal pattern in height, physical measurements and metabolism. This might lead to a better understanding of the total problem of mental subnormality. We want to know why many are smaller than normal, have a poor circulation and are excessively thin or obese. This may be the interest of paediatricians in the future, rather than the interest of the rare condition (Rundle 1970).

The main value of full investigation however is to the parents. Most people of average intelligence have a sense of the implications of scientific investigation. The realisation that the child's backwardness is caused by an abnormality which can be revealed by scientific means can dispel many mythical conceptions, such as 'bad blood' or 'sins of the parents'. Although still deeply and emotionally involved in the child's handicap, they can view it in the same light as a parent seeing a child handicapped by anterior poliomyelitis. In part it mitigates the feeling of guilt. A child with the broad thumb syndrome, Rubinstein-Taybi syndrome, was taken to see a well-known expert. The mother and child were treated with consideration, but the child was photographed and measured, his palm and foot prints were taken and blood was removed. One expected the mother to query the value of this and possibly to be upset. On the contrary it was found that she gained a deep-rooted satisfaction from the interest taken in her child, and realised that the experts attached no blame to her. Parents treated like this will not 'shop around' to see other doctors or ask for second opinions.

Place for Investigation

At the same time the essential utilitarian investigations, such as expert testing of sight and hearing and a psychological assessment, must take place. These investigations may be made when the child is either an outpatient or an inpatient in hospital. If he is recommended for physiotherapy, many of the tests and observations on him can be carried out when he attends for treatment. Although one would not advocate unnecessary separations from home, a period in hospital can be of great value for observation. Facilities in a children's ward in a hospital for the subnormal could be used. The staff and buildings are geared to deal with difficult children. The child can attend the 'school' for the severely subnormal run by the hospital authorities, and a report can be obtained from the school staff as to how he compares in development, speech and play with other mentally handicapped children. If the mother can stay in hospital with the child, she can be a witness to the interest taken in him and his visit can be made enjoyable.

Information to Parents

After the investigations the findings must be explained to the parents. If they are intelligent people it will be possible to give them an accurate resumé of the findings. If there is a chromosome abnormality the parents can be shown the photographs of the karyotype, and the abnormality can be pointed out and its significance discussed. If the condition appears to be due to an abnormal birth, the likely cause of damage to the brain, asphyxia, low blood sugar, can be discussed. With many cases there are several 'red herrings'. There may be a significant family history, an illness in the first six weeks of pregnancy, an abnormal birth, and a severe illness in infancy. The parents can be told the doubtful significance of any one of these causes. The value to the parents of being treated as intelligent people, able to discuss a scientific problem, is immense.

Genetic Advice

Most parents ask for genetic advice immediately they know of their child's backwardness. Even if they do not ask it should be mentioned as it is at the back of their minds. In some areas there are special clinics for genetic advice, but many parents would like to have advice from the paediatrician. With a chromosome abnormality, an up to date opinion of its significance can be obtained from the expert and relayed to the parents. In known recessive conditions the 1 : 4 likelihood of a similarly affected child can be explained. The parents will also want to know the likelihood of the normal siblings having an affected child. Dr. Fraser Roberts's advice (given verbally) applies to the siblings. 'They know their unpleasant gene. We do not know ours.' The parents can be told that they are in no worse a predicament about recessive inheritance than any one of us, unless they marry near relatives.

There is the more difficult question of advice to parents who have a single affected child with no clear aetiology. It is possible for these parents to have a second similar child, even when on occasions there has been the 'red herring' of a difficult birth to account for the condition. In the heterogeneous group of non-specific types, the overall risk of recurrence after a single affected child is of the order of 1 : 30 to 1 : 20. If two children are already affected, the recurrence risk approaches the 1 : 4 of a normal recessive condition.

SPECIAL CLINIC FOR THE MENTALLY RETARDED

After the investigations and early discussions, the parents cannot be left with their problems, and there is need for a regular follow up. This may be done at an outpatient clinic, but there is value in a special clinic for these children, run by someone especially interested in mental subnormality. The parents can then bring the child at intervals of about three months for general help and advice. Arrangements may have to be made to transport him. They will continue to discuss the aspects of the problem that have already been discussed with them. They will remember a distant relative with an abnormality and want to know the significance. They may want to ask about forms of treatment that have been mentioned in the family. They may want to ask advice on how to tell the in-laws, and how the affected child's presence will affect other children.

The clinic can be the referral point for the therapists treating the child. If there is a delay in reaching the milestones of movement, or the child has abnormal tone, or there is a danger of developing deformities, physiotherapy can be arranged. The parents need encouragement to put the child on the floor to play, and to help him with walking. If there are specific feeding problems, a motor speech defect or a language delay, the speech therapist can give help. At the clinic, the parents can be encouraged to talk to the child, and to respond to and encourage every communication, however basic, that he makes; and the work of the speech therapist can be supported.

The special clinic can be the centre for periodic reassessment. Reassessment is needed at regular intervals, both in the clinical and developmental areas. On the clinical side problems such as the first occurrence and control of fits arise. There may be a need to refer the child for a particular investigation. Nowadays it is considered justifiable to arrange heart surgery for a mongol with a septal defect. Every retarded child should have a physical reassessment annually. His development can be recorded at each attendance; and this may reveal disappointing lags and surprising improvement. One child, who had been known to a clinic from a few months of age, did not raise his head in supine until he was 22 months, and walked at 7 years. Yet he was able to live in a children's home and attend a school for the mentally subnormal, and later work in an adult work centre (figure 12.1). This progress was helped at all stages by physiotherapy and by stimulation from nursing staff. If there is a marked lag in normal progress it is necessary to ask why, and often a further psychological assessment may help.

It is of value if the doctor has some experience of adults with mental retardation. Doctors with access to a local authority training centre or a workshop in a hospital for the subnormal can show parents what an older child can do. A parent with a mongol child can gain reassurance by a visit to a workshop where mongols are assembling parts for television or making cement blocks.

The parents will ask questions such as 'Will he ever walk?' Experience shows that nearly all severely subnormal children walk eventually, if they are stimulated by being put on the floor to play and helped to pull themselves to standing, unless there is the added

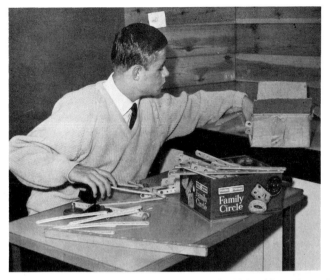

Fig. 12.1 A mentally retarded boy who did not raise his head in supine until 22 months of age and did not walk until 7 years old, but who later, as a result of stimulation and training, is able to do simple factory work.

complication of cerebral palsy. Some do not walk till 9 or 10 years of age or later, and then walk well as adults.

The other main question is, 'Will he ever talk?' It has been said that normal children of one year of age have a few words of speech. As few of these children have a mental age of less than one year, nearly all of them should have speech; and the majority speak in sentences.

Another query is, 'Will he ever do any useful work?' If a baby of 1 year is behaving like a 3–4 month old, it is generally fair to say that he will grow up to have an IQ of 30–40. At this level adults can do simple factory work, such as fitting clips on cards, and the parents can be told—particularly the parents of mongols—that this is the likely outcome.

PSYCHOLOGICAL ASSESSMENT

All mentally retarded children should see a psychologist. It is preferable if he can see the child at an early age, and several times before school age, to assess progress. Tests beyond the skill of the doctor are needed to get a full picture.

The Terman-Merrill and Merrill-Palmer tests may be helpful. If the child has an additional handicap such as blindness, tests specifically designed for the handicap should be used. Social maturity tests such as the Vineland or the Catell test may be used. Specific tests such as the Peabody test and the Reynell Language tests can pinpoint particular difficulties. All these tests give a report on the child's present ability. Other psychologists would test a handicapped child on a scale of tests adapted by Woodward from Piaget's concept of child's learning. By watching the child's play one can note his ability to learn and progress to the next stage of learning, e.g. a child of 12–18 months will obtain a toy that is out of reach by pulling the attached string; a child of 18 months can go further and can see how the string can be manipulated. These tests will show the level a much older mentally retarded child has reached in learning. It is felt that unless a child has reached an 18 month level, he is unlikely to benefit from play in a nursery school.

If the psychologist is brought into the assessment team, mistakes in diagnosis, such as misdiagnosing an aphasic or athetoid child, are less likely to happen.

THERAPEUTIC HELP

Physiotherapy

The movements of a mentally handicapped child may be abnormal in three ways.

1   His gross motor development may be retarded as part of the total delay in development. The majority of mentally retarded children are late in head control, sitting up, crawling and walking. There is a danger that after a period of pushing the child in these skills, the mother may give up and leave him lying in a cot. A physiotherapist can give encouragement and expert advice. Some of these children will not be ready to walk till 7 years or later; and unless changes of posture and attempts at mobility are encouraged before that age, the legs will become hypotonic, and contractures and deformities of the feet may develop which prevent later ambulation. There may be hypoplasia and osteoporesis of bones due to disuse. The child can spend part of the day lying supine on a wedge with toys in front of him. He can be put in a chair fitted with a tray

for toys. He can be supported to stand at a standing table for short periods, to develop balance reactions. Moving toys and trolleys or an infant crawler can be used. The use of walkers and baby bouncers is justified with these children if there is no cerebral palsy.

2 The delay in achieving normal movement may be due to cerebral palsy. These children need expert help, as described on pages 141–153. Passive methods, such as the Bobath techniques, must be employed at first. If encouraged many of these children will have the drive to pull themselves up and attempt walking. It is felt that this should not be discouraged in mentally retarded children, even if it may lead to a bad pattern of walking; cooperation in attaining a good walking pattern cannot always be obtained.

3 Some mentally retarded children are overactive. The motor ability is their greatest asset. Advice on suitable big safe toys and apparatus is needed for these children. They may require padded helmets on their heads if there is danger of falling.

Speech Therapy

The mentally retarded child is late in all the developmental stages of language development. Babbling is late. The production of sounds like 'g' and 'n'—a normal 9 month achievement—may be delayed for years; and actual words may not be spoken until 10 years or later. Even then, two word sentences may still be achieved. Preceding this slow formation of executive language, the understanding of auditory symbols and speech may be developing at a much slower rate than normal. A child of average intelligence understands words, sentences and commands for several months or years before he can say them himself. This gap between understanding and speech is very much longer in a mentally retarded child. A child may not understand 'bye-bye' until $2\frac{1}{2}$ years, and may not say it till 6 years old or later. These facts must be explained to parents. This does not mean that it is not worthwhile to stimulate the child to understand and speak, in exactly the same way as with a normal child; but the whole process will take longer. Parents must be encouraged to reward simple babbling with a smile of pleasure at whatever age it develops; and to practise playfully sounds like 'g', 'n' and 'bye-bye' at a much later age than is normal. Many parents may find this task embarrassing; but they need to be assured that this simple type of stimulation is very worthwhile, and has important end results. It will eventually lead to words and sentences. At the same time, the mother (and the family) must talk to the child in simple language as she washes and dresses him, explaining what she is doing and naming parts of his body and his clothes. It is important that she uses the same word for an object each time, e.g. 'coat', not 'mac' one day and 'cardigan' the next. It was found by Cashdan & Jeffree (1966) in a survey on mentally retarded children at home with their families, that after a time mothers ceased to talk to their mentally retarded child. In this way the development of language was further depressed. It is known that children in institutions speak later and understand later than normal children; but this situation may occur in a family home, unless the parents are supported. It is also found that all children learn speech from adults not from other children. They also learn speech close at hand, sitting on their mother's lap. Children do not respond at first to language shouted at them from a distance. Mothers must be encouraged to speak to their child close at hand.

It is in this setting that the speech therapist may help the mentally retarded. She may be needed to help with feeding problems and with dysarthria if the child has a movement defect. But in the realm of the mentally retarded her main task is one of language stimulation. She can develop auditory discrimination by helping the child to distinguish everyday sounds. She can encourage babble and copying intonation. She may help in selecting the most suitable vocabulary to use. Mein (1961) has drawn up a list of words used in conversation by subnormal patients, which may act as a guide to the type of vocabulary needed.

It is found that where a speech therapist is employed to encourage language, in the home, in the training school, or in a hospital for the subnormal, there is a spurt in the amount of language used by the children. Her presence on the staff emphasises to all the other care staff looking after the children the importance of speech.

If speech will never develop in a child, the speech therapist can encourage gesture as a form of communication (Levitt).

Training in Daily Living Activities

Parents with a handicapped child are usually totally unprepared to face the task of training one who will not make normal progress towards independence and must receive help. Some advice can be given at the special clinic. Often a social worker can visit the home and discuss all the problems. The person making these visits must have concrete advice to give if she is to be certain of acceptance on a domiciliary visit. She needs to have special knowledge on the type of help needed, and where it can be obtained. Part of her skills must be knowledge of suitable chairs for use at home, of push chairs such as the 'baby buggy' to take the child out, of suitable bowls and spoons to aid self-feeding, and of methods of teaching dressing with suitable clothes. She should advise on supplies of disposable napkins and on laundry services. There is a gap in this type of service, and ideally an occupational therapist should be asked to help too. She can visit the home and see how the parents manage with bathing and toileting. A social worker or a member of the therapy staff might find group sessions with mothers a means of giving support.

EDUCATIONAL PROVISION
FOR MENTALLY RETARDED

Schools for the Educationally Subnormal

The usual daytime provision for these children is at a special school or centre, at present called a School for the Educationally Subnormal in England and Wales. In some areas, children can start at the age of $2\frac{1}{2}$ to 3 years and can take part in a nursery school type of training. By the age of 3 years, the child may be physically active, without the understanding of a normal 3 year old. He may show the destructive tendencies of a much younger child. He may not yet understand even simple commands. At this age some mothers may be expecting another child. Daytime provision at the age of 3 years can be a great help.

In other areas, the child is admitted to the special centre at the age of 5 years and stays throughout his school life. The early emphasis is on training in social skills, such as feeding and dressing himself, and in constructive play (figure 12.2). Speech, language and manual skills are developed as fully as possible. In some cases, simple reading, telling the time and understanding money can be taught. These children can be taught cooking, woodwork and domestic tasks.

At school, as they are so often clumsy and awkward, particular

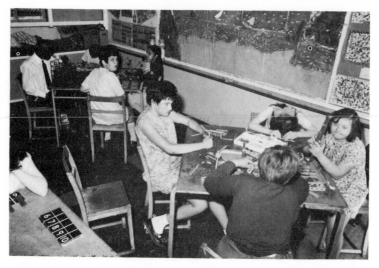

Fig. 12.2   Class of mentally retarded children in a training school.

emphasis is laid on training movement skills. It is considered that the children need to have a sense of their own body image. Many need to develop hand and finger skills, as the retarded often have flabby, awkward hands. The acquisition of clear and accurate speech with a use of language is emphasised.

The progress at school in daily living activity skills can be charted on a Progressive Assessment Chart designed by Gunzburg (1960) (figure 12.3).

This chart provides a visual check of progress in the four areas of self-help, communication, socialisation and occupation, and will pinpoint specific weaknesses in social development. Each space is numbered to represent a particular skill and is shaded in when this skill is attained—e.g.

Dressing   25   Cares for himself at the toilet and cleans himself
26   Brushes his teeth
28   Tidies hair at regular intervals

Further Education

Mentally retarded adolescents may go on learning after the age of 16 years, and often after the age of 20 years. Brand, Shakespeare &

Name _____   Age _____

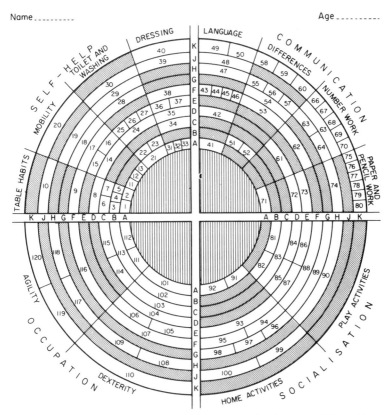

Fig. 12.3 Progress assessment chart of the social development of 'Mongol'
children (by kind permission of Dr H Gunzberg)

Woods (1961) have shown that some severely handicapped adults
can learn basic social skills, such as dressing themselves, that their
mastery of language can improve, and that skills in art and woodwork can develop. Quite a number of mentally handicapped adults
in the IQ range 45–60 can learn to do simple reading and arithmetic, to handle money and to tell the time, even as late as 30 years.
Possibly some of these people had been underestimated in childhood, but the value of education after 16 years has been noted in
schools for the physically handicapped and the deaf.

Special Care Units

There are children who do not fit into this type of centre, and they fall roughly into two types. First there is a group of hyperactive, distractible children, many of them epileptic and speechless, who are very difficult to control in a normal home. Although able to walk and run about, they tend to be of a very low intelligence. Some show autistic features. A special class is needed for them in any training school. The staffing needs to be in the order of at least two adults in a class of eight children. The emphasis is on social training, play and the use of large apparatus. Examples of the type of training are shown in the list of activities on page 215. The provision of a class of this type in any area will prevent the exhausted parents from requesting residential placement.

A second special class is needed for a group of children who are unable to walk and are severely physically as well as mentally handicapped. Many are cases of cerebral palsy due to birth injury, and have other handicaps such as epilepsy. Some are cases of spina bifida, with mental subnormality; and a collection of the rarer types of severe subnormality.

A list of the medical conditions in two special care units is given in table 12.1.

Table 12.1   Medical conditions in two special care units

Medical Condition	No.
Spastic quadriplegia	5
Spina bifida	4
Multiple congenital abnormalities	3
Down's syndrome with severe heart defect	2
Severe athetosis	2
Histidinaemia	1
Hypsarrhythmia	1
Suspected absent corpus callosum	1
Progressive condition	1
Occipital meningocele	1
Blind with cerebral abnormality	1
Spasticity and epilepsy following measles encephalitis	1
Spasticity and epilepsy following road accident	1

Training

In England there is at present no definite staff training to care for these two groups, who may be increasing in numbers. Work has been done by Morgenstern (1969) in the training of these severely handicapped children. They can be taught to recognise shapes and colours, to distinguish sounds, and to do constructive tasks such as putting pellets into a cup. After patient training, this may lead to an ability to do simple factory work.

Psychologists are currently working on a method of training called behaviour modification or operant conditioning (Skinner). The child is rewarded by a smile or a small sweet for every positive act, even as simple as attempting to take off a sock. Over a period, continuous reinforcement of this nature will lead to his being able to dress, and to other social abilities.

Activities with Special Care Unit Children
[adapted from Piaget]

1   Play with child with your own fingers. Touch him. Play with his fingers. Hide fingers. Hide hand.
2   Bulge out your face and burst your lips. Let child feel. Use facial expression.
3   Shine a torch and see if eyes follow. Play daily with this. Hide the light. Reveal it again.
4   Play at hand gestures.
5   Play with a handkerchief—carrying out all kinds of activities with it.
6   Hang toys (which make a noise when touched) immediately in front of child's vision when he is lying down.
7   Suspend toys near feet so that child has to try to stretch out to touch them.
8   Comb your hair closely in front of child. Put on cream, lipstick, etc. using a mirror. Wear a hat.
9   Pull out tongue.
10   Wear a poppet necklet.
11   At one and the same time hang a toy which makes a noise and a handkerchief on to a piece of string or elastic near the child's reach.
12   Sing daily and keep a record of songs sung.

13   Give the child different objects to handle—paper, tissue paper, shiny paper, cardboard tubes, cloth toys, plastic toys.

14   When toys suspend in front of child, move them with a long stick from different angles.

15   Hang ribbons of different colours.

16   Have a range of different sounds—bell in a ball, stone in a safe tin.

17   Play with sound, etc. the sounds in front of, behind, at the side of the child. A long way from him, near him. Call to him from different positions in room.

18   Carry or wheel child to several different positions in the room in any one day.

19   Play with a pan and a lid.

20   Get a stick and play at tapping different objects in front of the child, behind him, near him, far away, etc.

21   Get a cover and put over child. Repeat and respond to his actions. Now put over your head for him to pull off, over and over again.

22   Place small objects on palm of child's hand. Play giving and taking. Or just putting objects on palm if he lets go.

23   Encourage child to grasp different fingers on your hand. Bend on, waggle on, poke thumb, etc.

24   Play with a bandage. Let the child pull it out. Repeat with small ball of string.

25   Introduce bits of brightly coloured material on a string. Blow at them through a tube or fan them.

26   Play at opening and closing your fists in front of the child.

27   Put a mirror in front of him. Fix to table if he is sitting in a chair.

28   Pencil/stick play holding games.

29   Soft collar and belt introduced.

   This work could be undertaken by someone interested in child development. Operant conditioning may eventually lead to toilet training, and many will learn to feed themselves.

Day Hospital

Some of these children are so severely handicapped that hospital care is needed, and for these a day hospital attached to a children's hospital or a hospital for the subnormal would prevent a request for residential care. The children would return home to sleep. This applies particularly to the few cases of spina bifida, who, after surgery, are left with mental retardation, and also need attention for skin ulcers, care of the ileostomy and encouragement in the use of leg appliances and special wheel chairs.

Special Schools for Specific Handicaps

There is a tendency to place all mentally handicapped children of a particular age in one class, despite a mixture of handicaps such as blindness, deafness and cerebral palsy. Sometimes this means that it is difficult to obtain specific help for a particular handicap. It is hoped that in selected cases the arrangement by which children with a handicap are educated in a special school dealing with that handicap will be extended to the severely subnormal.

The Cerebral Palsied Child

One group are children with cerebral palsy. There are a certain number of cerebral palsied children in the IQ range 40–60 who cannot benefit from the education provided in schools for the physically handicapped, but who have considerable potential for learning and later sheltered employment. They may have the specific handicaps of cerebral palsied children, such as perceptual problems, problems of space discrimination, visuomotor and apraxic difficulties, dysarthria, high frequency deafness, and receptive and executive communication disorders. These difficulties cannot be dealt with in a special care unit or in an ordinary class in a training school. The numbers in any area do not appear to be great. Possibly a special class in a school dealing with cerebral palsied children of higher intelligence, where the know-how of staff working with these children can be utilised, would be the correct placement. In England the Spastics Society have opened a resident school, Meldreth Manor School, near Cambridge, for this special group of cerebral palsied children of low intelligence. It is hoped that the research and the methods used at this school will pay dividends, and the knowledge gained be widely disseminated.

The Blind Child

Another group requiring special training are the blind mentally subnormal. In the developed countries, childhood blindness is a comparative rarity; but when it occurs it is often associated with a cerebral defect, and the majority of blind children are of subnormal intelligence. Blind and partially blind children do not fit into normal training schools, where the type of training is mainly visual, and special units are needed. Because of the numbers, any special training must be in a resident setting during the school years. The incidence is in the order of 2–3 children of this type in a population of 200,000. Some will be too severely retarded for special training. England and Wales have at present four units of this type.

There is also a need for day units or residential units for the deaf-blind postrubella children, many of whom function as severely subnormal.

Behaviour Disorders

There is a particular group of mentally subnormal children who are difficult both to treat and to place. This is the group of children with severe behaviour disorders which appear to be organically determined. Some are extremely hyperactive, distractible, often epileptic, and destructive to their surroundings. They wreck an organised class, and need to be continuously watched at home or in a centre. Doors must be locked, or they will rush out and get injured, lost or even drowned. They will climb to very unsafe heights. Most hospitals for the subnormal have a few of this type, and they may grow into interfering aggressive adults, usually unemployable. Some are severely subnormal, unable to speak or understand. Others may show evidence of an intelligence at an educationally subnormal level.

A second group with severe behaviour disorders are withdrawn, self-mutilating, taking little notice of people or their surroundings. They appear to want to return 'in utero', hiding themselves under beds or in cupboards. They may become aggressive if attempts are made to break their routine.

Any special units to give these two groups of children therapeutic help and training by methods such as behaviour modification would need a staffing ratio of more than one staff to one child.

Few such units exist. Elsewhere these children must be contained in a play environment, such as an adventure playground, which is safe for themselves and where they cannot damage other children. The play should be interspersed with periods of individual help from an occupational therapis, teacher, nurse or dedicated untrained person. Drugs such as chlordiazepepoxide, diazepam, chlorpromazine and haloperidol have a place in treatment. There is a danger of overuse of drugs with mentally retarded children, and the medication given should be kept under close supervision.

Resident schools may be the only practical solution for these groups of doubly handicapped children; but it is hoped that they will have a boarding school life comparable to that of normal children. They should have normal school holidays, and if possible go home for weekends.

Short-Term Resident Care

Facilities for short-term resident care is often requested by parents where children live at home. This is needed to give the family some relief from full time care and should be arranged in a suitable children's home. For some children holiday camps could be arranged.

Permanent Resident Care

Resident care for children may be requested for medical or social reasons. The reasons which make parents ask for permanent resident placement are many.

Medical or Psychiatric Reasons 1 The child may be physically handicapped and require total nursing care.
2 Epilepsy may be so serious that normal family life is impossible.
3 The behaviour problems may be severe. He may be hyperactive, doing dangerous actions such as turning on gas taps. He may be destructive, tearing his clothes or breaking windows. He may develop unacceptable habits, such as exposing himself or openly masturbating. He may become noisy and truculent, and too much for a mother on her own to cope with.

Social Reasons 1 Illness or death of the member of the family looking after the child.

2 Illegitimacy.

3 Family disharmony due to the presence of a handicapped child.

4 A mild behaviour problem such as unacceptable eating habits.

5 In other cases the family may make a well thought out decision to find a resident place, because it is felt that it is best for the family, that the adolescent will have a fuller life, and that it is better to make an arrangement before the parents die.

These decisions are social ones, and should never be made in a hurry.

In the first set of circumstances, the correct placement would be a medical one, presumably in a hospital or medically orientated institution. In the second set the decision is a social one, and the placement should be a home or hostel run by social services in the community.

Hospitals for the Subnormal

These large institutions still form the backbone of the resident care of the subnormal in England and many other countries. They have come in for a considerable amount of criticism. They are considered too large (700–2000 beds). The buildings may be poor, the staff inadequate, and the location too far from the child's own home for contact to be maintained. There may be frequent changes of staff, and the patient does not have the security of one person responsible for his care and training—a mother figure for him. The hospital staff may be too authoritarian in their attitudes and the patients may not have enough say in their own lives, such as choosing their own clothes and maintaining them. They may be underoccupied and understimulated. The environment for long stay patients may be too medically orientated. Possibly they should not be called 'patients', or be looked after by nurses, under the overall charge of doctors.

Many of these accusations are justified; but these hospitals can be happy places, and the patient may be well known as a personality in his own right. Many hospitals could be considered similar to village communities, with school, workshops, shops, laundry, administrative buildings, recreational hall, chapel, swimming pool, gardens and sports fields. A resident may have more freedom than in his own home, where he cannot move around his own town freely. For a severely handicapped person, there may be more of interest going on than if he was chairbound in his own home. In a fairly large community it is easier to arrange films, dances and activities at the mental level of the residents.

There is a danger that large institutions become institution orientated rather than patient orientated. The needs of staff and staff careers may take precedence over the need to give the patients the fullest life possible. There should be plenty of small rooms, bright and attractive furniture, individual colour schemes around each bed, and bedrooms of one to four beds rather than large dormitories, with plenty of room for personal possessions.

Hostels or Children's Home

The vast majority of severely subnormal children could live in more home-like surroundings than are usually provided in a hospital for the subnormal. This has been proved by experience in Sweden and Denmark, and in some areas of Britain. Kushlik (1967) has shown that units for up to 25 children in the centre of the community of about 100,000 will provide all the resident places for children that are needed. The child can live near the family home and have frequent contact with normal urban life. He can attend the local training school daily and have the advantage of going out into the community. In this way these handicapped children will not be 'put away', but will lead as near a normal life as possible and grow up to be socially acceptable.

Later Work Opportunities

With more opportunities for training and education as children, the majority of mentally subnormal adults are now found to be able to do useful work in a sheltered environment. They can work in laundries and kitchens. Work can be found for them on farms. There are numerous simple tasks in industry which cannot be done by machinery, and are ideally suited for the mentally subnormal (figures 12.4 and 12.5).

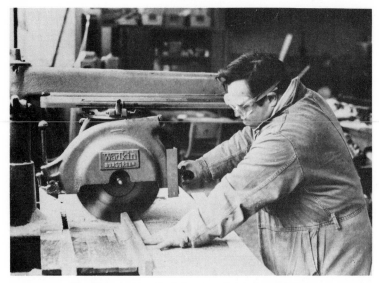

Fig. 12.4 A mongol adult using electrical equipment.

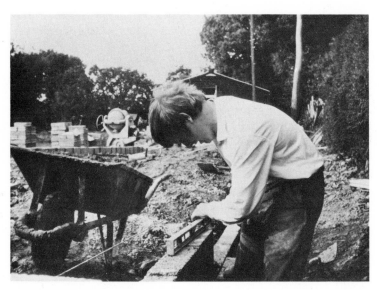

Fig. 12.5 A mongol adolescent boy laying bricks and using a spirit level. (By kind permission of the National Society for Mentally Handicapped Children)

REFERENCES

Brand J, Shakespeare R & Woods G E (1969) Psychological development of the severely subnormal after 16 years of age. *Dev. Med. Childh. Neurol.* **11**, 783

Cashdan A & Jefree D M (1966) The influence of the home background on the development of severely subnormal children. *Brit. J. med. Psychol.* **39**, 313

Clarke A D B & Clarke A M (1965) *Mental Deficiency. The Changing Outlook.* Methuen, London

Grunewald K (1969) Norms for the planning of 13 institutions for the mentally retarded. *Changing Patterns in Residential Services for the Mentally Retarded, 1968.* Board of Health and Welfare, Stockholm, Washington

Gunzburg H C (1960) *The Social Rehabilitation of the Subnormal.* Bailliere, Tindall & Cox, London

Kushlik A (1967) The Wessex Plan for evaluating the effectiveness of residential care for the severely subnormal. *Proceedings of the 1st Congress of the International Association for the Scientific Study of Mental Deficiency, Montpelier*

Levitt L M A (1970) *A Method of Communication for Non-Speaking Severely Subnormal Children.* The Spastics Society, London

Loring J (1966) Meldreth (Cambs.) a pioneer unit for training spastic children. *Spec. Educ.* **55**, 20

Loring J & Mason A eds. (1968) *Proceedings on a Seminar on Mental Handicap with Special Reference to Cerebral Palsy.* Spastics Society, London

Luria A R (1963) *The Mentally Retarded Child.* Pergamon, Oxford

Mein R (1961) A study of the oral vocabularies of severely subnormal children. *J. ment. Def. Res.* **5**, 52

Merren E, Macauley M & MacMillan M (1965) Teaching severely retarded children to walk. *Dev. Med. Childh. Neurol.* **5**, 549

Mittler P (1972) *Learning Processes in the Mentally Handicapped.* Educational Research in Great Britain. University of London, London

Morgenstern M, Beer H L & Morgenstern F (1966) *Practical Training with the Severely Handicapped Child.* Heinemann, London

O'Connor N & Hermelin B (1963) *Speech and Thought in Severe Subnormality.* Pergamon, Oxford

Primary Progress Assessment Chart (PPAC) SEFA (Publications), Birmingham

Shakespeare R (1971) *The Psychological Assessment of Mental Handicap,* ed. Peter Mittler. Methuen, London

Skinner B F (1957) *Verbal Behaviour.* Appleton Century Crofts, New York

Stephen E & Robertson J (1966) Can institutional care improve? *Spec. Educ.* **55**

Stevens M (1972) *The Educational Needs of Severely Subnormal Children.* Arnold, London

Tizard J (1964) *Community Services for the Mentally Handicapped.* Oxford University Press, London

Williams P (1969) Child care and mental handicap. *Dev. Med. Childh. Neurol.* **11**

Woodward M (1962) The application of Piaget's theory to the training of the subnormal. *J. ment. Subnorm.* **8**, 17

Chapter 13
The Child with Learning Difficulties

In classes at normal primary schools there are a number of children—variously estimated as between 3% and 10%—who have difficulty in mastering the basic skills of reading, writing and arithmetic. They can be grouped from a clinical angle into nine categories:

1 Mentally severely subnormal child, IQ under 50
2 Sensory impaired child with defects of sight or hearing
3 Severely physically and neurologically impaired child
4 Speech retarded child

These four categories have been dealt with in other chapters. It is hoped that nowadays their disabilities will have been noted before 5 years of age and appropriate educational placement arranged.

5 Educationally subnormal child
6 'Clumsy' child, often described as a child with 'minimal cerebral dysfunction'
7 Dyslexic child—the child with a specific difficulty in mastering reading
8 Hyperactive, distractible child
9 Emotionally disturbed child—not considered specifically in this book

The clinical problems in categories 5, 6, 7 and 8 are considered below.

EDUCATIONALLY SUBNORMAL CHILD (ESN)

These children have an IQ between 50 and 70, but they should, with help, be able to master the three Rs and to learn socially acceptable behaviour. They should later earn their living and live an independent life.

The author studied the medical conditions in 200 of these children attending one special school for the educationally subnormal, and the findings are given in tables 13.1–13.10. They emphasise the large number of clinical conditions found in schools and classes for the educationally subnormal.

Cultural Pattern

There was a higher than normal incidence of social class V; but 70% of the children had fathers with professional, managerial, skilled or semi-skilled manual jobs. This finding is contrary to the generally accepted belief that ESN children come almost exclusively from social class V.

Table 13.1   Social Class of 188 ESN Children

Social Class	No.	%	% Incidence in Borough
I	3	1·6	5·5
II	5	2·7	14·3
III	99	52·7	57·6
IV	25	13·0	14·8
V	56	30·0	7·8
	188	100·0	100·0

Among the 56 children from social class V parents, there were five prematurely born children, one epileptic child and two with congenital abnormalities, suggesting a multifactorial cause for the backwardness in some of these socially deprived children.

In only 17% of the children was it felt that the low intelligence was a cultural and social pattern with no evidence of brain pathology.

Clinical Conditions

Genetic Causes

In 12.5% of the children, there was a possible genetic inheritance of the condition. In eight families (16 children) there were two siblings where both parents were of average or above average intelligence. Some of these children were clinically abnormal, with abnormal facies, microcephaly or low placed 'bat-ears'. All tests for abnormal amino acids in the urine were negative. Two brothers had delayed sexual development, and cytogenically showed elongation of one arm of the Y chromosome. These children must be considered cases of recessive inheritance of an as yet unexplained genetic condition.

Table 13.2   Dominant and Recessive Genetic Conditions

	No.
Dominant Inheritance	
Dystrophia myotonica (mother affected)	1
Von Recklinghausen's disease	1
Muscular dystrophy—female heterozygote (father affected)	1
Communication disorder (mother affected)	1
Abnormality of jaw (father and siblings affected)	1
Friedreich's ataxia	1
	6
Recessive Inheritance	
Cleft palate	1
Treated case of phenylketonuria	1
Abnormal renal condition (strong family history of ESN intelligence and congenital abnormalities)	1
Two ESN siblings in one family	16
	19

Congenital Abnormalities (9%)

Table 13.3   Congenital Abnormalities

	No.
High palate, abnormal shaped head, micrognathos, accessory auricles etc.	9
Multiple congenital abnormalities	3
Cleft palate, absent auditory meati, partial hearing loss	1
Down's syndrome	1
Amsterdam dwarf—Cordelia—de Lange syndrome	1
Prader Willi syndrome	1
Congenital heart defect	1
Arrested hydrocephalus (aqueduct stenosis)	1
	18

Birth History

Table 13.4   Birth Order of 187 Cases

Order	No.	%	Average % for country at 7 years (Pringle, Butler & Davie 1966)
1st	56	29·7	9·2
2nd	43	23·3	36·2
3rd	39	20·9	25·9
4th	24	12·8	14·7
5th	10	5·3	6·9
6th +	15	8·0	7·1
	187	100·0	100·0

There was a higher than normal incidence in first-born children from a high birth rank order.

Table 13.5   Abnormalities of Pregnancy, Birth and Infancy in 187 Cases

	No.
Abnormal pregnancy (rubella 1, shingles 1, hyperthyroidism 1, severe vomiting 2, severe APH 1)	6
Premature ($5\frac{1}{2}$ lb and under)	28
Postmature (over 2 weeks)	3
Over 10 lb birth weight	6
Surgical induction for rhesus antibodies	1
Pre-eclampsia and/or abnormal birth with postnatal illness in child	19
Twins (all, also premature)	5
Illness after Birth which Appeared to Account for Condition	
Tuberculous meningitis	2
Fits in infancy followed by hemiplegia	2
? Diabetes	1

In 63 (31·5%) children, one or other of these birth complications was present. The possible effect of prematurity was emphasised by Drillien (1964), who states that 'there is a marked excess of dull, retarded and defective children in those under $4\frac{1}{2}$ lb at birth, particularly if there were adverse factors in the environment'.

Early Milestones

Table 13.6   Age of Walking in 179 Cases

Age	No.	
1 year	35	
12–18 months	63	
18–24 months	38	
24–30 months	33	
30–36 months	4	
36–42 months	4	43
42–48 months	1	
Over 48 months	1	
	179	

Forty-three children could be considered abnormally late in walking.

Table 13.7   Age of Saying First Words in 172 Cases

Age	No.	
1 year	41	
12–18 months	21	
18–24 months	37	
24–30 months	30	
30–36 months	5	
36–42 months	26	43
42–48 months	4	
Over 48 months	8	
	172	

Forty-three cases (not the same children as those late in walking) could be considered late in saying the first words.

Table 13.8 Age of Saying Two to Three Word Phrases in 173 Cases

Age	No.
18–24 months	1
24–30 months	61
30–36 months	21
36–42 months	23 ⎫
42–48 months	8 ⎪
48–54 months	13 ⎬ 90
54–60 months	23 ⎪
Very late	23 ⎭
	173

Ninety were late in talking in sentences. This observation was specifically mentioned by many parents and was often the first indication to them that their child might be intellectually retarded, although not mentally severely subnormal—IQ under 50.

Clinical Examination

Table 13.9 Percentile for Height (Tanner–Whitehouse Standard)

	%
97	1·6
90	5·9
75	11·3
50	24·3
25	17·7
10	17·7
3	8·6
Below 3	12·9
	100·0

The general height of these children was below average, and twenty-three were exceptionally small, being below the third percentile. The short stature appeared more obvious in the older children and is illustrated by the fact that although the children stayed at school until over 16 years of age, the tallest child in the series was 5 feet $8\frac{1}{2}$ inches. In a normal school, some six footers would be expected.

Table 13.10   Cranial Circumference (Martin 1925)

	%
More than 3 standard deviations above normal	1·5
3 SD above normal	6·3
Normal	27·0
3 SD below normal	56·1
More than 3 SD below normal	9·2

The head circumference was well below average in 65·3% of these children.

Eye Defects

Forty-two children (21%) had abnormal eye conditions and in twenty-three children this was a refractive error. Gardiner (1969) found visual defects in 25% of children in a resident school for ESN children. Two children had cataracts. Eighteen children had defective eye movements. Some had a simple strabismus. In a number of children the eye movements were uncoordinated, or there was a field of vision defect suggesting a cerebral lesion.

Hearing Defects

Twenty children had been reported as having a hearing loss at some period in their childhood. The hearing loss was often associated with an upper respiratory infection in a socially deprived child. It is difficult to assess the importance of a period of hearing loss on eventual intellectual and language development. Three children were severely deaf and wore a hearing aid.

Language Defects

It has been noted that many educationally subnormal children are late in speaking in phrases. There were seven children who were abnormally late, and in these cases a communication disorder, receptive or executive aphasia, could be diagnosed. Two were siblings in a family where the other two siblings were severely retarded, and there was one child whose mother was an intelligent woman with similar executive difficulty. Five of these children also had a motor speech defect.

Neurological Examination

There were four children with hemiplegia, three right and one left, and one boy with spastic diplegia.

There were 24 cases who would come under the umbrella of 'minimal cerebral dysfunction' or 'minimal brain damage' (Walton 1963, Illingworth 1963). The abnormal neurological signs included abnormal eye movements, motor speech defects and dribbling, increased reflexes, marked associated movements in the hands at an older age, perceptual and body image defects noted by the teacher and physiotherapist, astereognosis, disinclination to use a hand, inability to hop and pes cavus. Many in this group were hyperactive. Thirteen had a history of birth abnormality or a later illness involving the brain, and of these thirteen, three were epileptic. Four were epileptic of the eleven children without a significant history.

There were twenty-two epileptic children among the 200 children, the majority having infrequent fits.

Twenty-eight were clearly left-handed.

Behaviour Disorders

Rutter and others (1970) in the Isle of Wight study stated that 'emotional and behavioural disorders are much commoner in intellectually retarded children, in particular hyperactivity, distractibility and lack of concentration'. These disorders might be a sign of severe emotional disturbance, but in most cases appear to be organically orientated, and are often associated with a positive history of neurological illness, epilepsy or an abnormal EEG. This group are difficult to incorporate into the classroom situation, but with small classes, and specially trained teachers, the problems these children show seem to decrease as they get older, and are less in evidence among older children.

Management of ESN Child

Preschool Help

Children who will later have an intelligence within the range 50–70 show evidence of retardation before the age of 5 years. They should be fully investigated as soon as a delay in reaching milestones pinpoints a possible abnormality. In diagnosing mental retardation in early life, the paediatrician should be aware that the child, although retarded, may not be severely subnormal. The prognosis for later life is much better if the child is in the IQ range 50–70.

Various forms of therapy may help these children in the preschool years. Physiotherapy may encourage motor skills, and the child's awareness of his own body. Some authorities (Tansley 1960) think that it is important that these children early establish a fixed dominance of either the right or the left side. Attendance at a 'language-delay' class may be arranged. Attendance at a nursery school may be of benefit.

Educational Placement

Possibly these children should be referred for special educational placement early. A period of frustration and failure, competing with more intelligent children, can be prevented. Placement in a special class in a normal school may be preferable to placement in a special school, but classes should be small, and the staff trained in modern methods of approach to teaching disabled children.

Therapy in School

The services of a physiotherapist should be available during school life. She should treat a fair number of children regularly, and maintain a 'watching brief' over uncoordinated, clumsy children with poor gait who need her help. There is a place for an occupational therapist. Many of these children need individual help with daily living activities, such as learning to dress, tie laces and cut out with scissors, and often with basic skills such as independent toileting. Delay in achieving skills is often due to specific visuomotor difficulties. It was felt in some children that early help could have prevented later problems in holding down a job. A speech therapist is needed in any school dealing with these children. The language problems are so great that a school for the educationally subnormal should have a full-time therapist on the staff.

Drug Treatment

All epileptic children should receive medication, and if a midday dose is prescribed, there should be responsible staff at the school to give the medicine to the child. A secure place must be provided for storing the drugs. Some children are prescribed drugs for hyperactive or distractible behaviour. Doctors prescribing these drugs should be in constant contact with the child's teacher, to make sure that the drug is having the desired effect, and is not unduly depressing school performance.

Adolescence

In the survey described in this chapter, it was found that the organic problems noted in early school life assumed less importance as the child got older, as a result of the early help in many fields. The majority of the children left school to go straight into employment, and a minority required further training.

THE CLUMSY CHILD

(Child with minimal cerebral dysfunction)

This concept has grown out of the work with cerebral palsied children. For some years teachers in normal schools have noticed children who were conspicuous because of awkward movements and learning problems. Many were referred, via the school medical officer, to clinics for cerebral palsied children, with a suggestion that the child appeared 'spastic'. It was interesting to find that in a high proportion of these children, unknown to the teachers, there was a history of a premature or abnormal birth or a factor in the child's medical history which might cause 'brain damage'. Workers such as Prechtl (1962) followed up children who had survived an abnormal birth with neonatal complications. In a proportion of them there was a later incidence of motor incoordination and overactive behaviour. Prechtl described a 'choreiform' syndrome in these children.

Learning Difficulties

It is found that clumsy children often have other difficulties apart from disorders of movement. Some show a motor speech defect. Others have a language delay. They may have difficulty in finding the right word and may use a small vocabulary for their age. There may be evidence of receptive or executive dysphasia. Children with this type of defect may also find it difficult to learn to read.

They may have difficulties in drawing and writing, due either to motor incoordination or, more often, to a visuomotor problem. A child's effort to draw a man may be quite bizarre for his chronological and mental age. The picture shown in figure 13.1 was drawn recently in a clinic by a child of 7 years 9 months, who was able to read. He was quite satisfied with the drawing. Arithmetic ability

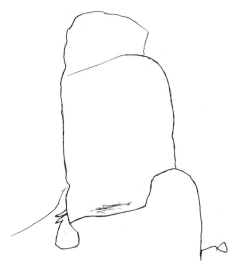

Fig. 13.1 An attempt to draw a man by an 8 year old boy who had mastered simple reading, but had severe perceptual difficulties.

may be poor. These children may show the learning problems that have been noted in those with a clear diagnosis of cerebral palsy, such as inability to copy shapes or recognise pictures, to dress themselves or to recognise distance.

Coupled with motor incoordination and learning problems, the child may show hyperactivity, lack of concentration and distractible behaviour.

Early History

Many intelligent parents have worried about their child's abnormal development before the age of 5 years and have tried to obtain specialised help early. Usually the child's problems are noted outside the family for the first time by the school teacher.

Problems in School

The abnormalities that teachers may recognise are listed below (Bowley 1969):
1 Generally *restless* and overactive
2 Generally *clumsy* and awkward in movement
3 *Everyday skills*
  Slow to tie up shoelaces
  Slow to button up coat
4 *Use of tools*
  Inaccurate in hammering nails
  Lacks skill in cutting with scissors
5 *Writing*
  Has very untidy handwriting
  Reverses letters or parts of words
6 *Reading*
  Is making poor progress in reading for his age
  Reverses words or letters when reading, e.g. on/no
7 *Speech*
  Does not speak clearly
  Shows hesitancy in speech
8 *Drawing*
  Has difficulty in drawing a man showing related parts
  Has difficulty in copying a simple geometric shape

9   *Physical education*
    Can seldom catch a ball
    Frequently trips over small obstacles
    Unable to hop

Neurological Examination

Sight and hearing must be tested.

Many of these children show minimal signs of neurological involvement. These can be divided into what have been called 'hard' and 'soft' signs.

Hard Signs

1   Incoordinated eye movements
2   Excessive dribbling, swallowing and chewing difficulties. Dysarthria
3   Defective hearing, particularly a high frequency loss
4   Minimal cerebral palsy. Evidence of
mild athetosis with defective hand movements
minimal hemiplegia
minimal spasticity with a tendency to plantar flexion
ataxia with delayed balance reactions
5   Abnormal signs such as extensor plantar response, a tremor, or an incoordinated finger-nose test
6   Congenital abnormalities, such as abnormally shaped skull or low placed ears
7   Amino acid or chromosome anomalies. Children with phenyl-ketonuria, non-ketotic hyperglycaemia, or Turner's or Klinefelter's syndrome may present as awkward incoordinated children with learning problems
8   An abnormal EEG

Soft Signs

1   Poor posture and gait
2   Body image difficulties shown by difficulty in dressing or assembling pieces of a doll
3   Gerstmann's test, showing an inability in a child older than 9 years to recognise which finger is touched when he is blindfold
4   Strabismus

5   Delayed speech development
6   Associated movements, e.g. in a child older than 9 years: when he is asked to clench one hand, he automatically clenches the other
7   Fog's test. If the child stands on the outside of his feet, he automatically adopts an abnormal posture of his hands
8   Right-left confusion
9   Hand function skills below the child's age as shown by the scales suggested by Rosenbloom (1970)

Psychological Assessment

After the neurological examination the child must be referred for a psychological examination. His motor abilities may be observed either by the clinician or by the psychologist using the Oseretzky Test of Motor Ability, which gives norms for motor skills up to the age of 16 years.

Other tests used are:
WISC Performance and Vocabulary Scales
English Picture Vocabulary for Verbal Comprehension
Illinois Test of Psycholinguistic Abilities
Reynell Language Test
Frostig Perception Tests
Bender/Gestalt Designs
Reading Age
Arithmetic Age

Difficulties in perception and in the areas of visuomotor, auditory-memory or auditory-discrimination skills may be pinpointed.

Management and Help

After a full clinical and psychological assessment, there must be a team discussion among all members of the staff dealing with the child to decide what specific help he needs. It may be physiotherapy, speech therapy and/or occupational therapy. Often specific training is needed from a remedial teacher. This can be given on an individual basis or in a small remedial class attached to a normal school. Training in perceptual skills, as suggested by Frostig, can be used. The parents must fully understand the child's difficulties and learn to accept them in the home situation or the learning problems will be overlaid by emotional problems.

DYSLEXIA

A child is considered to suffer from dyslexia, or difficulty in mastering reading, if he is at least two years retarded in reading despite an
average intelligence.

Types

There may be a *history of dyslexia* in the family, particularly among
the males. The father, although adequately supporting the family,
may be a non-reader or unduly slow in reading. He is doing a job
which does not require this skill. A son today with this handicap
will not obtain the examination success required to hold down any
but a manual job. It is suggested that there is an inherited inability
to interpret the meaning of verbal symbols and to correlate the
word with its appearance in print. The affected child has usually
been late in talking; and there is a history of early unintelligible
speech. If the child learns to read he will be a poor speller. On
psychological testing, the performance scores will be higher than the
verbal scores, and the child will show difficulty in auditory memory
and discrimination.

A child with *minimal cerebral dysfunction* may present as a child
with dyslexia, although many of these children have no difficulty
with reading. There is likely to be an early history suggesting brain
'damage'. The child shows other learning difficulty and some of the
'hard' and 'soft' neurological signs described in the previous section.
In these children, the overall verbal skills may be higher than the
visuomotor and performance skills. They may have difficulty in
scanning a line of print, and reading words in the correct order, and
they may also be very poor in drawing, writing and arithmetic.

There are a group of children with reading difficulties due to
adverse social and emotional circumstances. This is likely to occur in
social class V where the language used by the parents to the child is
primitive and consists mainly of negative and positive commands. It
occurs particularly in children who have been deprived of close
contact with adults in an institution or in hospital. These children
have not had sufficient language experience to be ready for reading
at the right age.

Some children have difficulty in mastering the method used to teach reading at their particular school, either a visual or an auditory method.

Management

Children 'at risk' of having difficulties in learning to read may be found by a survey on those with speech problems under 5 years. The speech therapist helping a child with defects of auditory memory may help him in his first attempts with reading; and work with dyslexic children is included in the training of some speech therapists.

During school life these children should be identified and classified early and given help individually or in small remedial

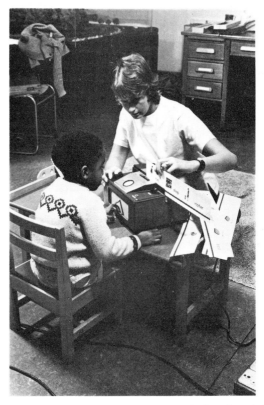

Fig. 13.2   A Language Master being used by a speech therapist to help a child with language delay to see a picture, hear and read a word, and hear his own attempt at speaking the word.

classes. A different approach to the method of teaching reading may
be all that is needed. Children with specific problems need help in
the particular area where they have difficulties, visual or auditory
memory. A teacher, psychologist or occupational therapist may
help with perceptual training, on the lines suggested by Frostig.
A speech therapist may join the team to help children with auditory
or language problems. A teaching machine, such as a Language
Master, which emphasises the written word by picture and by
speech, can be used (figure 13.2).

   With specific help the results can be good, but without this help
children will be handicapped in the labour market and there may be
an overlaid behaviour problem which can lead to later withdrawal
or delinquency.

THE HYPERACTIVE CHILD

The hyperactive or hyperkinetic child is well known to teachers and
psychologists. The problems in the classroom usually necessitate
some form of special education. The hyperactive child appears to
have difficulty in sorting out the many sensory stimuli reaching him
from his environment. Because of this, he must immediately respond to every stimulus he meets. As a result, he is distractible and
lacks the power to concentrate. On seeing a picture, he notices every
visual clue and is unable to sort out the essentials. He also responds
to every auditory clue, and has difficulty in bringing his attention to
bear on the principal auditory stimulus, such as the teacher's voice
in the classroom. He is hyperactive in a motor sense, and must get
up and investigate every sound or sight he hears. He cannot adapt
negatively to the inessential.

Early History

In the majority of these children, there is an early history of possible
brain pathology. A high proportion are epileptic, and others have
an abnormal EEG recording. The restlessness and hyperactivity
may have been noted early in the child's life and have been a cause
of sleep and feeding problems. Difficulties in management occur at
an early age and there is danger of rejection by the parents, family
friction and emotional problems in the child.

Management

Placement in a nursery school may give relief to the mother, but is not necessarily the right type of management for the child. A free and lively permissive environment gives him no training in controlling his stimulus bound behaviour.

These children require play and education in a structural environment. Cruikshank (1967) has advocated education in rooms which have opaque windows and no pictures on the walls. The teacher is expected to dress very simply. In this type of environment, the child is taught to concentrate on a particular task and to learn to master his difficulties.

The children as a group must be taught in small classes with a structured curriculum and individual sessions in a small bare room may be helpful. Schools for the educationally subnormal require facilities to deal with children of this type. There is a need for some school places for children under 5 years.

Drug Treatment

Tranquillizing drugs have a place in treatment. Phenobarbitone usually accentuates the condition and should not be prescribed. Amphetamine in large doses may have a marked effect, although it may be due to the fact that the drug is producing a depression.

REFERENCES

BAX M & MACKEITH R (ed.) (1963) *Minimal Cerebral Dysfunction.* Heinemann, London

BIRCH H G, RICHARDSON S A, BAIRD D, HOROBIN G & ILLSLEY R (1970) *Mental Subnormality in the Community.* Williams & Wilkins, Baltimore

BOWLEY A (1969) Reading difficulty with minor neurological dysfunction. *Dev. Med. Childh. Neurol.* **11**, 4, 493

CRUIKSHANK W M (1967) *The Brain Injured Child in Home, School and Community.* Syracuse University Press, Syracuse

DEPARTMENT OF EDUCATION AND SCIENCE (1972) *Children with Specific Reading Difficulties.* HMSO, London

DOYLE P J (1962) The organic hyperkinetic syndrome. *J. Sch. Hlth.* **8**

DRILLIEN C (1964) *The Growth and Development of the Prematurely Born Infant.* E & S Livingstone, London

FOG E & FOG M (1963) Cerebral inhibition examined by associated movements. *Minimal Cerebral Dysfunction.* Heinemann, London

FRANCES-WILLIAM J (1963) Problems of development in children with minimal brain damage. *Minimal Cerebral Dysfunction*. Heinemann, London

FROSTIG M, LEFEVRER D W & SHITTLESEY J R B (1961) *A Developmental Test of Visual Perception*. College of Special Education, London

GARDINER P (1969) *Aspects of Developmental and Paediatric Ophthalmology. Clinics in Developmental Medicine*, No. 32. Spastics Society & William Heinemann, London

ILLINGWORTH R (1963) *Minimal Brain Damage. Little Clubs in Developmental Medicine*, No. 10. Heinemann, London

KEPHART N C (1964) *The Slow Learner in the Classroom*. Charles Merrill, Ohio

KINSBOURNE M & WARRINGTON E K (1963) A study of finger agnosia. *Brain* **85**, 47

LEWIN R S (1963) *The Brain Injured Child*. National Society for Crippled Children and Adults, Chicago

MCDONALD A (1965) *Gestational Age, Size and Maturity. Clinics in Developmental Medicine*, No. 19. Spastics Society & William Heinemann, London

MCDONALD CRITCHLEY (1964) *The Dyslexic Child*. Heinemann, London

MONEY J ed. (1962) *Reading Disability*. Johns Hopkins Press, Baltimore

NAIDOO S (1972) *Specific Dyslexia*. Pitman, London

PRECHTL H F R & STEMMER C J (1962) The choreiform syndrome in children. *Dev. Med. Childh. Neurol.* **4**, 119

PRINGLE M L K, BUTLER N R & DAVIE R (1966) *11,000 Seven Year Olds*. Longman, London

ROSENBLOOM L & HORTON M E (1970) The maturation of fine prehension in young children. *Dev. Med. Childh. Neurol.* **13**, 13

RUTTER M, TIZARD J & WHITMORE K (1970) *Education, Health and Behaviour*. Longman, London

STRAUSS A A & LEHTINEN L E (1947) *Psychopathology and Education of the Brain Injured Child*. Grune & Stratton, New York

TANNER J M (1960) *Education and Physical Growth*. University of London Press, London

TANSLEY A E & GULLIFORD R (1960) *The Education of Slow Learning Children*. Routledge & Kegan Paul, London

TOUWEN B C L & PRECHTL H F R (1970) *The Neurological Examination of the Child with Minor Nervous Dysfunction*. Heinemann, London

WALTON J (1963) *Minimal Brain Damage. Little Club Clinics in Developmental Medicine*, No. 10. Heinemann, London

Chapter 14
Defects of Speech and Language. Autism

It has been realised in the last twenty years that delayed acquisition of speech, and more fundamentally a lack of development of comprehension, are two handicapping conditions which require special education. These defects may occur in a multiple handicapped child, but they can occur as superficially a single handicap. Three resident special schools for speech disorders have been opened in England and many schools taking unusual handicaps, such as the Rudolf Steiner Schools, are also providing special facilities for these children. There is a need for more school places and considerably more provision is made in the USA. Common speech disorders are classified in table 14.1.

Surveys on Language Delay

Several surveys have been carried out on delayed speech and the incidence of speech defects in children. In the study of 1000 children in Newcastle-upon-Tyne in 1964 it was found that at 3 years 9 months 18% of children had some form of defect (table 14.2).

In a recent survey (Butler, Peckham & Sheridan 1972) on 15,496 seven year old British children it was found that at this age between 10% and 13% (according to the observer) had some speech defect, and 1·4% had a marked speech defect. There were twice as many boys with a speech defect as girls, and there was a significant trend towards a lower social class and a higher birth order. The children with speech defect showed more clumsiness and visual defects and 32·4% of them were non-readers.

Criteria for Referral for Special Help

It can be said that to understand and to speak is as important for normal development as to see and to hear. An inability to speak normally will prevent a child from taking part in normal education

Table 14.1   Classification of the Common Speech Disorders in Childhood

---

1   Disorders of voicing (dysphonia)
  With demonstrable disease of the larynx
  Without demonstrable disease of the larynx

2   Disorders of rhythm (dysrhythmia)
  Clutter
  Stammer or hesitation

3   Disorders of articulation with demonstrable dysfunction of articulatory apparatus (dysarthria)
  Due to neurological abnormalities
   Cerebral palsy
   Suprabulbar palsy
   Lower motor neurone lesions
  Due to local abnormalities

Jaws and teeth	Hypomandibulosis
	Other malocclusion
Tongue	Tie
	Tongue thrust
Lips	Cleft lip (only)
	Other
Palate	Cleft (with or without cleft lip)
	Other
Pharynx	Large pharynx (palatal disproportion)
	Acquired disease
Mixed	

4   Disorders of articulation without demonstrable dysfunction of articulatory apparatus (secondary speech disorders)
  Secondary to hearing defect
  Secondary to mental retardation
  Secondary to psychogenic disorders
  Secondary to dysphasia due to brain damage

5   Developmental speech disorder syndrome (specific developmental speech disorders)
  Involving language development and articulation
  Involving articulation only

6   Mixed cases

7   Unclassified and other

Table 14.2 Survey of Speech Defects in 1000 Children in Newcastle-upon-Tyne (1964)

Type of defect	No.
Delayed development of speech	5
Resolving defects of articulation	95
Severe persistent defects of articulation	44
Defective articulation and stammering	37
	181

and an inability to understand will prevent the child from developing an inner language.

Children on the 'at risk' register should be watched to make sure language is developing normally, but it seems likely that a number of children with language delay will be missed if reliance is placed only on the 'at risk' register and a complete survey of all children for language development should be the responsibility of the Medical Officer of Health (table 14.3). Perhaps this is a task that is ideally carried out by a health visitor, who goes into the home and can hear the child speak in his normal environment. She can listen to any worries the family have about speech development.

Table 14.3 Criteria for Referral of Children with Language Delay (Renfrew 1972)

Age	Symptom
2 years	Saying no words
3 years	Saying no more than single words, or is unintelligible to the family
4 years	Unintelligible to strangers, or is stammering frequently
6 years	Speech difficulties are drawing attention to the child

Referral

If any of the heading in table 14.3 apply to a particular child he should be referred to a paediatrician. His hearing should be efficiently tested in both ears. There must be a full developmental assessment.

Developmental tests such as those devised by Sheridan (1968) are helpful. The paediatrician can ascertain if the child has developed normally in the areas of Posture and Large Movements; Vision and Fine Movements; Social Behaviour and Play. A specific delay in speech development, with skills in other areas up to the normal for the child's age, makes it unlikely that mental retardation is the cause for the delay in acquisition of speech.

History

Details of the pregnancy, birth, neonatal period and any subsequent illnesses must be obtained. On questioning, one may find that there is a family history of speech delay and/or a difficulty in learning to read. There may be an incidence of left/right confusion, and delayed acquisition of a dominant hand in members of the immediate family.

Examination

After one has gained the confidence of the child, the inside of the mouth must be examined. Conditions such as tongue-tie or enlarged tonsils are very unlikely to be the cause but it is possible that a cleft palate or submucous cleft has passed unnoticed. The hard palate may be high or the soft palate may be unduly short, preventing nasopharyngeal closure.

A neurological examination of the cranial nerves may reveal defective movements of the tongue, lips, palate and facial muscles. Evidence of other neurological deficits may be noted in examining the reflex state, gait, posture and movements.

Investigations such as EEG examination, aminoaciduria and chromosome investigations are indicated in quite a number of cases. Children with phenylketonuria and histidinaemia have presented as developmental aphasia.

In cases presenting primarily as a speech defect or a language delay, the child should be referred to a speech therapist.

Speech Therapist's Examination

The application of specific tests to analyse a speech problem is the province of a speech therapist. In certain centres in Britain and other parts of the world the training of speech therapists has become a university degree course. Speech therapists learn about the use of tests which involve speech and language development, and their expertise in this field covers some areas of clinical or educational psychology.

Assessment of Understanding of Speech   Normal babies begin to understand simple speech from 8 months of age onwards; but there is a gap of several months or a year before the child speaks the words himself. 'Pat-a-cake' is understood by a baby of 10 months, but he may be aged 18 months to 2 years before he says the words. In mentally retarded children the understanding of simple language is markedly delayed and the gap between understanding and speech is much greater than is normal.

To ascertain why a child is not speaking, it is essential to find out first how much he understands.

The Peabody Picture Vocabulary Test is used for children from the age of 21 months upwards. The child is asked to point to one of four pictures corresponding to a word spoken by the examiner.

The Reynell Test is used to test the comprehension of simple and complex sentences by the use of simple toys. It can be used for severely physically handicapped children who can signify their understanding of a command by 'eye pointing'.

Assessment of Spoken Language   The Reynell Test also gives an estimate of the child's ability to use speech by asking him to name objects and to describe actions and pictures.

Tests by Renfrew take this examination still further. Her tests pinpoint the difficulties in verbal expression of older children, particularly those who are educationally subnormal.

Auditory Discrimination   Children with delayed language may have specific difficulties. The child may have difficulty in analysing sounds and turning them into meaningful language. A child may hear a sound and be unable to distinguish which sound he hears. The condition has been considered comparable to colour blindness.

To test ability in auditory discrimination, the child is shown pictures of objects whose names sound alike. Incorrect selection often indicates that he is not distinguishing slight differences.

Auditory Memory An ability to remember and repeat sounds is essential to the development of language. The child is asked by the therapist to repeat random numbers or a sentence planned in an unusual way. The speech therapist, with her knowledge of speech development, can note his difficulties.

Illinois Test of Psycholinguistic Abilities With this test the child's specific language difficulties are analysed. The use of the test can show the examiner the child's ability:

to understand simple questions—auditory decoding
to comprehend pictures—visual decoding
to make an auditory-vocal association
to understand visual symbols
to express his ideas in words—vocal encoding
to give appropriate gestures—motor encoding

Speech therapists and psychologists can use this test to analyse the particular difficulty in marked language delay and to indicate the age level the child has reached in each ability.

Articulatory Difficulties Whilst carrying out the preceding tests, the speech therapist can analyse the child's articulation. She will note how he imitates sounds and syllables, and how many phonemes or speech-sounds he uses. He may use only 20 instead of the usual 40. She can also notice the distortions which he uses, and any difficulty he has in voice production. There may be problems of phonation due to vocal cord abnormalities. A recent test of articulation has been developed in Edinburgh (1971).

Speech Organs The speech therapist will be the expert in noting minor motor speech difficulties. She will examine the movements of the face, lips, tongue and palate, and the control of respiration. She will test the ability to suck and swallow, and to chew vertically and horizontally. She will notice whether the child dribbles unduly. She will also test his awareness of his tongue and lips, and his capacity to carry out movements on command, as there may be an element of apraxia in his speech difficulties. She will also test his ability to make sensory discriminations with his lips and tongue, and will find out whether he can distinguish hot and cold on his lips. She will note if the various muscles are used correctly in eating and in speech.

Use of Language   The speech therapist can ask questions and test the child's ability to give information by the use of speech. She can listen to his use of grammar and to his efforts at telling a story.

Other Findings   In cases of pure language delay, it is important to have a report on the home circumstances from a social worker. In some families, the delay is due to the fact that parents are not talking to their children and television may be to blame. It is known that children learn early speech from adults and not from other children. Children brought up in institutions are 'at risk' of a language delay.

Referral to Other Specialists

It may be necessary to refer the child to an ear, nose and throat consultant for his opinion, particularly if there is dysphonia. A neurological opinion may be needed.

Diagnosis

After a full investigation and discussion with other workers, the speech therapist can give a report on her findings. She will be the expert to tell the paediatrician whether the speech need cause any worry; whether it can be cured by simple advice to the mother; whether a change in the social environment, such as admission to a nursery school, is desirable; whether she can help the child by taking him on for periods of speech therapy; and whether he has a speech disorder which will constitute a severe handicap and require special education.

HANDICAPPING SPEECH DEFECTS

The handicapping speech defects which will require special education are listed below. They may be divided into seven types. Defective hearing (dealt with in chapter 3)

Congenital abnormalities—cleft lip and palate
Articulation difficulties. Dysarthria
Articulation and language difficulties. Executive aphasia
Articulation, language and comprehension difficulties. Receptive
  aphasia and mental retardation
Articulation, language, comprehension and communication
  difficulties. Autism
Psychogenic disturbance. Elective mutism

Cleft Lip and Palate

These congenital deformities can only be included under the overall
heading of the physically handicapped child in so far as the child's
speech is affected. A child may be born with:

a   Submucous cleft. There is a defect in the midline of the bony
palate and the muscular layer of the soft palate. The defect is closed
by mucous membrane.

b   Median cleft involving the uvula or soft palate.

c   Median cleft involving the hard and soft palate, and which may
extend to the alveolus.

d   Lateral clefts of one or both sides which involve the lip (harelip)
as well as the palate.

e   Incomplete varieties of lateral clefts.

f   The most severe deformity, which involves a bilateral cleft,
leaving a small piece of skin in the premaxillary portion of the
alveolus. The premaxilla may be separated from the maxilla on both
sides and project forward.

The deformity can occur in association with other abnormalities,
such as cerebral defects, mental subnormality, abnormalities of the
eyes, congenital heart defects and chromosome anomalies. The
child with this deformity needs a full assessment. The condition may
occur in association with micrognathus, as in Pierre Robin
syndrome.

Developmental Problems

Feeding   This may be difficult due to a leakage of milk into the
nasal cavity in the case of a cleft palate, or, in the case of a harelip, to
an inability to suck.

Speech If a child has a defect in the muscles of the palate, due either to a submucous cleft or to a patent cleft in hard or soft palate, he will be unable to achieve oronasal closure between the palate and the pharynx. Air will escape into the nasal cavity during speech and the speech will have a nasal quality. An immobile upper lip, or an inability to make good apposition with the lower lip, will cause difficulty in articulating sounds such as 'p', 'b' and 'm'.

Upper Respiratory Infections Because of the deformity, the child is more liable to upper respiration infections and there is a danger of superadded middle ear deafness.

Management

Surgery The cleft in the lip is usually closed at about 3 months of age.

The optimum time for repair of the cleft palate is a matter for argument. It should certainly be repaired before speech begins. If the child develops an abnormal speech, he also develops an abnormal auditory and kinaesthetic feedback from his own speech and this may be difficult to correct later. It is felt by some surgeons and speech therapists that 6 months of age may be an ideal time if the child is fit. Others will postpone operation until 18 months. Where it has been impossible to close the palate completely, an obturator may have to be worn in the mouth.

In cases of severe deformity further cosmetic operations may be necessary. Orthodontic treatment may be required if the teeth are crowded.

Speech Therapy Speech therapy is often unnecessary after successful surgery; many children will correct bad patterns of speech that have developed. If the child is not speaking clearly, and in particular if nasal speech persists, speech therapy may be given after 4 years of age.

Genetic Advice

The overall 'at risk' figures of further affected children are as follows.

Harelip with or without cleft palate

Subsequent siblings, parents normal	1 in 25
Subsequent siblings, one parent affected	1 in 10
Children of affected person	1 in 30

Median cleft palate

Subsequent siblings, parents normal, no relatives affected	1 in 50
Subsequent siblings, parents normal, another relative affected	1 in 10
Subsequent siblings, one parent affected	1 in 6
Children of affected person	1 in 50

Dysarthria

Speech defects of this type occur in children with cerebral palsy. The speech defect is a spasticity or athetosis of the muscles used for speech production; and it occurs in between 30% and 70% of all cases of cerebral palsy. There are disturbances of respiratory control, disturbances of voicing (dysphonia), disturbances of rhythm (dysrhythmia) and disturbances of articulation (dysarthria). There may also be a dyspraxia. These speech defects are discussed under cerebral palsy.

In two conditions there is a motor disorder of speech with minimal or no evidence of cerebral palsy.

Congenital Pseudobulbar Palsy

Cases of this condition are seen in schools for speech disorders and unfortunately in hospitals for the subnormal, and are likely to present at assessment centres for full investigation.

The syndrome was originally described by Worster Drought (1956). In his original description he considered that the condition was due to impaired development of the pyramidal tract nerve fibres above and proceeding from the motor cortex to the cranial nerve nuclei which supply the muscles of articulation. The condition can be associated with a spastic hemiplegia. Some cases are due to birth abnormalities.

In the complete syndrome, the child shows weakness or paralysis of the tongue (even protrusion being absent), paresis of the lips, an inability to round the lips and a marked paralysis of the soft palate, which may hang down like a curtain or be very short. Nasopharyngeal closure is impossible. The child is unable to speak, although his comprehension may be good. He is a persistent dribbler. Milder manifestations of the syndrome may be seen.

Drugs have little effect on the dribbling. Operations for removal of the salivary glands are not desirable, as the condition is due to an inability to swallow the saliva, and not due to excessive formation. Surgery has left a dry mouth and a liability to decay of the teeth.

The swallowing in select cases may be dramatically helped by a pharyngopalatal push back operation. It is suggested that the paralysed palate prevents the child from being able to push the saliva back into the nasopharynx, and a pool of saliva collects between the base of the tongue and the palate. Operation on the palate may enable the child to swallow the saliva. Where there is paralysis of the tongue, he can be taught to suck and then swallow the saliva.

The condition may be associated with normal intelligence but there may be a superadded aphasia. In a hospital for the subnormal, one boy who had had no schooling taught himself to read all the patients' names on the hospital files. After surgery his dribbling improved so that he was able to work in a laundry but he never learnt to speak.

These children need special help in a school for speech disorders. Their numbers are too small for special classes, and they could not take their place in a normal class.

Mobius Syndrome

This condition was first described by Mobius in 1892. There is total or partial facial palsy presumed to be due to an agenesis of cranial nerve nuclei. The child cannot smile or raise his eyebrows, and his face is flat and expressionless. There are swallowing, sucking and dribbling difficulties, and a laryngeal stridor and a dysphonia. The condition may be due to an interference in development of the mandibular and hyoid arches; but it has been described associated with other congenital abnormalities such as absent fingers and deformed limbs.

Executive Aphasia

A child with executive aphasia may have a mild difficulty in understanding language, and may be below the average for his age on the Reynell Comprehension Test. He will show little or no speech at 3 years and in severe cases no speech when starting school. The inability to express himself will cause frustration and temper tantrums. Because he can understand, a child with this difficulty is likely to be able to fit into the family life and join in other children's activities better than the child with the more severe difficulty of a receptive aphasia. He appears to have an inner language.

Aetiology and Examination

These children are likely to be referred to an ear, nose and throat surgeon. Tongue-tie or enlarged tonsils may be blamed, but cannot be the cause.

There may be a family history of language delay and a confusion in laterality.

If there is a history of perinatal difficulties or a severe illness in childhood with neurological involvement, there may be minimal neurological signs suggesting a cerebral pathology.

Management

Children who have this specific difficulty need specialised help. They need training in a language delay class or a special school. Some of them are unfortunately placed in classes with children who are globally mentally retarded, when the language development is likely to be further delayed. Children with executive aphasia should have specific help from 3 years of age.

Receptive Aphasia or Dysphasia

'Aphasia is a breakdown in the comprehension and formulation of words giving rise to a disturbance of thought and a disorder of language' (Morley 1965). There may be a marked receptive or expressive component; and where the difficulty is only partial the word dysphasia is used.

Children with this difficulty cause concern to their parents early in life. Babbling may have been normal, but there may be little or no acquisition of normal baby words. The child shows motor skills up to the level of his age group and can crawl, climb, walk and feed himself at the norm for that milestone. He (and these children are usually male) manipulates the household appliances and mechanical toys at a normal age, and may be able to recognise pictures. The author knew one child with this difficulty who had an obsession for bath-plugs. At the age of $2\frac{1}{2}$ years he immediately pointed out the bath-plug in an advertisement of bathing equipment for the handicapped which happened to be in the examination room.

The parents early realise that the child is not understanding language at the level for his age. The question of a hearing loss is immediately raised, but by watching their own child, parents repeatedly have evidence that he can hear quiet sounds. He will respond immediately to the ice cream bell or father's car approaching.

In extreme cases the child may not comprehend even these sounds, but tests such as evoked response audiometry will demonstrate that he can hear. At the other end of the scale a receptive dysphasic child may understand simple commands at a level much below his age. A boy of 9 years, with average performance scores, had an understanding on language testing at a $2\frac{1}{2}$ year level.

Almost without exception, receptive aphasic children will show behaviour disorders. Their inability to understand may lead to marked hyperactivity and distractibility. Yet it can be shown that with a favourite mechanical task they are able to concentrate well. The frustration may lead to destructiveness and aggression towards other siblings and the situation in the family may be difficult to handle. With some children the condition of a severe delay in understanding language may present as autism but the fact that the child can organise his visual world suggests a different emphasis in the diagnosis. He should be referred to a paediatrician before 3 years of age.

Aetiology

There may be a family history of delay in speech development and in acquiring reading and writing skills and the child may be an extreme example of a dominant ill-defined genetic condition. There may be a history of late acquisition of a hand dominance or cross laterality in other members of the family.

Some cases follow an abnormal birth and evidence of perinatal birth trauma. Others follow an infective illness in childhood. Worster Drought (1971) described a group of children with a form of dysphasia following an encephalitis.

Examination

Careful observation should rule out mental retardation. Auditory testing may cause confusion, as a number of receptive aphasic children have a mild hearing loss which is not severe enough to account for the lack of understanding of spoken language.

A neurological examination may show evidence of minimal neurological deficits. The child may be clumsy in his movements and there may be an apraxic element in his speech and motor difficulties.

Management

If the delay in understanding speech is causing behaviour disorders, or the discrepancy between verbal and performance skills is marked, it is not safe to assume that the condition will correct itself.

It is also not sufficient to apply the remedy that is so often suggested: admission to a nursery school with normal children.

These children need specific help, and help is best given by individual speech therapy or attendance at a specially organised 'language delay' class. A small group of similarly affected children are taught a normal vocabulary step by step. For example, they may learn to distinguish hot and cold by feeling appropriate objects and repeating the words. They must learn nouns and verbs for each object and action. Too much pressure will immediately lead to a behaviour breakdown and the training must go very slowly. Often simple games in the class help to reinforce language. A speech therapist, psychologist or nursery school teacher may be interested in taking part in these classes. Possibly one or two of these classes are necessary in any population of 200,000. They have been set up in areas such as Bristol and Hounslow, London, and they are much more common in the USA.

A child with receptive aphasia is without a means of communication, which is essential for normal human development. There are two other methods of communication which can be used apart from speech—gesture and writing. Gesture and sign language should be allowed and gesture by the adult to the child can be used to augment an understanding of the word spoken.

Special Schools

If a child has evidence of intelligence and performance skills within the normal range, and a severe delay in understanding or acquiring language, admission to a special school for language disorders may be indicated. At these schools the child can be taught to communicate by learning to read and write. Lea (1970) at Moorhouse School for Speech Disorders has shown how these children can get a concept of nouns, verbs and other parts of speech by using written words in different colours for different parts of speech: red for nouns, blue for verbs and so on. Communication by writing is thus developed and the child can also be taught to use finger spelling.

In some children progress in speaking will be rapid. Others may acquire speech but later show problems in reading, writing and arithmetic. Others may never acquire a good understanding of speech and may never speak.

Adults

If these children are not diagnosed and treated early the eventual outcome may be very poor. In hospitals for the subnormal there are a number of adult patients (nearly always men) who are the skilled workers in the hospital workshop; and yet have no speech and little understanding. Six men of this type were noticed at one hospital. It was felt very strongly by staff that some of them could have achieved outside employment if help had been given early. They could have been taught reading, writing, measurement and many other educational skills. A description of one of these men follows.

'He was born on 27 April 1937. His early history is not known. He was admitted to hospital for tuberculosis at the age of 22 months and stayed until he was 7 years and 10 months. On discharge it was stated that he had never eaten solids, he did not speak but screeched like an animal, and he could not walk except by holding a chair. He was admitted direct to a hospital for the subnormal. He walked at 8 years but never spoke. He made his wants known by gestures. He attended hospital school and was said to be able to scrub floors and do jigsaw puzzles at 14 years. He worked in an Industrial Therapy Unit for many years.

He is a well-built man who makes contact with everybody he meets by incoordinated vowel sounds and gestures. At the age of 28 years he has been heard to make recognisable words such as 'Nother one'. X-ray of the skull, and chromosome and aminoaciduria investigations are normal. The EEG shows rather a featureless low amplitude record with no definite abnormality.'

The speech therapist's report states: 'Frederick is very excitable and shouts a lot—his shouting is incomprehensible. He is able to carry out commands if they are repeated several times, but he does not appear to understand questions. In fact he pays little attention to speech unless the volume is increased. Frederick vocalises a great deal—mainly using single syllables. However, he does sometimes use a recognisable word, 'Bye', 'Hello', and he is able to imitate simple words such as 'bed', 'car', 'man' fairly well. The speech musculature is mobile and control is poor. This applies particularly to the lateral movements of the tongue. The palate does not move in phonation and the speech is nasalised.'

His hearing appears to be normal, but he lacks comprehension of anything but the simplest commands.

Psychological report: An early Stanford–Binet test at the age of 12 years gave him a mental age of 2 years 11 months.

When reassessed for this study at the age of 31 years his executive speech was developmentally assessed at around a 13 month level; he did not score on the Peabody Test, but he probably understood one or two very simple commands.

On performance tests, however, he scored at a much higher level. WAIS Block Design and Object Assembly gave scaled scores of 2 and 7, giving a prorated IQ of 65. On the Hickey–Nebraska ('deaf' norms) Learning Ages ranged from 5 to 10 years with a median of $6\frac{1}{2}$ years, he scored an IQ of 58 on the Progressive Matrices, and his drawing of a man scored at a $6\frac{1}{4}$ level.

A repeated Stanford–Binet test gave him a mental age of 2 years 11 months, though the range of passes and failures was very wide and he passed tests up to the 7 year level.

This man is the outstanding worker in the Industrial Therapy

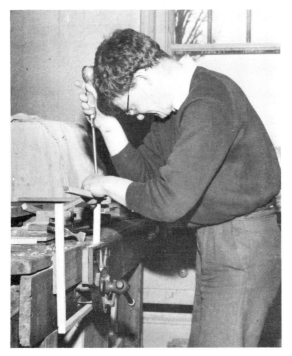

Fig. 14.1   Man described in the text with no speech and little understanding of speech, who is able to use electrical and carpentry equipment. He could be considered as suffering from a receptive and executive aphasia.

Department. With instructions carried out mainly by gesture and example he can quickly learn complicated tasks. He can safely and accurately use machines such as electrical drills (figure 14.1).

Autism

This subject comes under the overall umbrella of a speech defect: first, because this condition in any child would be revealed by the screening criteria suggested by Renfrew (1972); secondly, because all these children have a language defect; and thirdly, because modern thinking suggests that the condition is due to a defect in the child's ability to use and analyse his auditory and visual input. In fact some workers would consider autism as a more profound and disorganising form of receptive aphasia.

History

Heller (1908) first described a condition of dementia infantilis. The
children he described showed normal development until 2–3 years
of age, and then deteriorated to the level of idiocy. Kanner (1943)
described children with a condition he called infantile autism. The
child had a lack of affective rapport, appeared to be detached,
lacked emotional contact, showed overt failure to develop speech or
had a pedantic bizarre type of speech. Kanner laid emphasis on the
cold personalities of the parents of these children, and suggested
that their 'emotional' frigidity had led to the emotional withdrawal
of the child.

   Soon after Kanner's work was published, children who answered
his description were noted in increasing numbers. Many were found
in hospitals for the subnormal. To define the condition more
accurately, a working party was set up in London under the
chairmanship of Dr Mildred Creak. The condition was then called
the 'schizophrenic syndrome in childhood'. The Working Party
enunciated nine points. It stated however that each child with the
condition might not show all the characteristics; but it laid considerable importance on the ninth point.

1   Gross and sustained impairment of emotional relationships with
people. This includes the more usual aloofness and the empty
clinging (so called symbiosis); also abnormal behaviour towards
other people as persons, such as using them impersonally. Difficulty
in mixing and playing with other children is often outstanding and
long-lasting.
2   Apparent unawareness of his own personal identity to a degree
inappropriate to his age. This may be seen in abnormal behaviour
towards himself, such as posturing, or exploration and scrutiny of
parts of his body. Repeated self-directed aggression, sometimes
resulting in actual damage, may be another aspect of his lack of
integration (see also point 7), as also the confusion of personal
pronouns (see point 7).
3   Pathological preoccupation with particular objects or certain
characteristics of them, without regard to their accepted functions.
4   Sustained resistance to change in the environment, and a striv-
ing to maintain or restore sameness. In some instances behaviour
appears to aim at producing a state of perceptual monotony.
5   Abnormal perceptual experience (in the absence of discernible

organic abnormality) is implied by excessive, diminished or unpredictable response to sensory stimuli, e.g. visual and auditory avoidance (see also points 2 and 4) and insensitivity to pain and temperature.

6   Acute, excessive and seemingly illogical anxiety is a frequent phenomenon. This tends to be precipitated by change, whether in material environment or in routine, as well as by temporary interruption of a symbiotic attachment to persons or things (compare points 1, 2, 3 and 4). Apparently commonplace phenomena or objects seem to become invested with terrifying qualities. On the other hand, an appropriate sense of fear in the face of real danger may be lacking.

7   Speech may have been lost, or never acquired, or may have failed to develop beyond a level appropriate to an earlier stage. There may be confusion of personal pronouns (see point 2), echolalia or other mannerisms of use and diction. Though words or phrases may be uttered, they may convey no sense of ordinary communication.

8   Distortion in motility patterns, e.g. excess as in hyperkinesis; immobility as in katatonia; bizarre postures, or ritualistic mannerisms, such as rocking and spinning (themselves or objects).

9   A background of serious retardation in which islets of normal or exceptional intellectual function or skill may appear.

When used in everyday practice this list was too comprehensive. In fact the majority of children with mental retardation, even children with Down's syndrome, could come under the overall umbrella of this ill-defined condition.

Since then, other workers have added their own criteria. Clancy, Dugdale & Rendle-Short (1969), working in Australia, have suggested that the child can be diagnosed as autistic if he shows at least seven of the following fourteen criteria:

Great difficulty in mixing
Acts as deaf
Strong resistance to any learning
Lack of fear about realistic dangers
Resists change in routine
Prefers to indicate needs by gesture
Laughing and giggling for no apparent reason
Not cuddly

Marked physical overactivity
No eye contact
Unusual attachment to a particular object or objects
Spins objects
Repetitive and sustained odd play
Standoffish manner

Description of Condition

Yet, in spite of the difficulty of definition, the type of child who is described as autistic is well-known to workers with retarded children. He appears perfectly normal in physical features, body-build and gross movements of walking, climbing and manipulating toys. After being a quiet baby in early childhood, he has not appeared interested in his surroundings. He has not smiled or shown pleasure when seeing his mother. His early babble has soon ceased and has not progressed to simple words. He does not appear to understand speech, although there are frequent indications that he can hear. He will suddenly quieten if he hears a noise. Walking may be somewhat late, but is usually achieved by the normal progression from rolling over to crawling. The child takes little notice of people and concentrates his vision instead on objects which he plays with endlessly, such as a piece of string. From early childhood he becomes extremely distressed by any change in his environment.

Some children who must be considered mentally retarded never get beyond this stage. They do not understand speech, fiddle endlessly with the same object, scream if their routine is disturbed and often scream purposelely. They learn to feed themselves but never become toilet trained, and end up as the most difficult patients in a refractory ward of a hospital for the subnormal.

Some less affected children develop speech late and the speech may be inappropriate and echolalic. They appear out of touch with their environment and will take no notice of what is going on, and then suddenly repeat a sentence which might be considered at a normal level for their age. They may show evidence of a good memory. A child like this, without being able to communicate, may develop a motor skill such as going down a slide and even learn to take his place in a queue. Their movements, though agile, may be bizarre, walking on tip-toes, flapping their hands and flicking their fingers. Screaming attacks, aggressive episodes and an inability to recognise danger make later management difficult.

The condition may be a continuum, and the more intelligent children with this condition may learn to read and take a special interest in music or art, but remain detached and affectless.

One child aged 5 years, known to the author, took no notice of the proceedings at a Christmas party, and did not go up for a present when called for by Father Christmas. She suddenly screamed when seeing the ballons and for a time was uncontrollable. She then went past a car and said correctly the car number, SHU 350, showing that somehow she had learnt letters and numbers, but it would be impossible to incorporate this type of child into a normal class.

The condition is no longer considered as a form of schizophrenia. The adolescents and adults who suffered from infantile autism do not present as schizophrenia in adult life; there is no increased incidence of schizophrenia in the near family, and no evidence of hallucinations in the child.

The incidence is 4·5 per 10,000 school children in the population. The condition appears to occur equally in boys and girls.

Aetiology

Parents   It is now generally accepted that frigid, emotionally cold parents are *not* the cause of the condition. The parents are capable of having a normal warm relationship with their other children. The lack of rapport with the autistic child can cause a breakdown in the normal mother-child relationship; and the mother may secondarily be disturbed and insecure in any dealings with the child.

There is however, unexplained evidence that the parents more often belong to social classes I and II than the average in the community. Children who are socially deprived and institutionalised are more likely to show attention seeking behaviour.

Genetic Influences   There are occasional incidences of two affected children among a family of otherwise normal children.

Occasionally a child with a receptive aphasia and no autistic features, and a child with florid autism, occur in the same sibship. Either child may show a mild hearing loss.

Organic Causation   In the original description of autism, it was suggested that the condition began during infancy in a previously normal child. Careful scrutiny of cases reveals that the baby caused concern by undue quietness, undue fretfulness, feeding difficulties, delay in early speech sounds and other milestones from the first few months of life. The evidence for a sudden onset of the condition is not very strong, unless the condition followed a known illness such as encephalitis, or the child was later found to be suffering from a deteriorating neurological condition.

Prenatal Factors An occasional case has appeared to be due to an abnormal biochemical condition such as phenylketonuria. A chromosomal abnormality such as the XXXY anomaly has caused a condition indistinguishable from autism in a child. It is impossible to assess the importance of other prenatal factors.

Perinatal Factors An abnormal birth has been an antecedent in as many as 50% of cases of severe infantile involvement and a markedly premature birth may be a factor in the history.

Later Illness Some children have developed symptoms indistinguishable from autism following a febrile illness which was presumably an encephalitis. A high percentage of the severely affected children became epileptic in adolescence, and a large number show varying types of EEG abnormality. A raised blood lead content has been found in some children. This might be causal and account for the onset of the condition in later infancy when a child started to chew objects that unfortunately contained lead.

Undoubtedly autism is given as the diagnosis in children who are later found to have a deteriorating neurological condition. This has accounted for the deaths in later childhood of so-called autistic children who have deteriorated both in behaviour and function.

Types of Autism

Some workers would distinguish three types:
1   The autistic, profoundly retarded child. This condition is almost invariably found to be organic in origin.
2   The autistic child of normal intelligence. There are usually no indications pointing to an organic origin; and children in this group may improve considerably.
3   Children with apparently similar symptoms in which the condition develops after 11 years of age. These children will turn out to be cases of adolescent schizophrenia.

Nature of Autism

Psychologists consider that autism is a breakdown of sensorimotor integration. There is a failure in the central processing of incoming and outgoing material. There is also a profound receptive aphasia and the autistic child is unable to process auditory symbols. The defect may be so severe that he may develop no inner language and will not even use gestures. This distinguishes him superficially from the profoundly deaf child. His appreciation of sound may be limited to the bodily sounds he makes himself, such as grinding his teeth and snapping his fingers.

A less profoundly affected child may develop echolalic speech which he uses inappropriately. He may describe himself as 'You'. A severely subnormal child such as one with Down's syndrome, if asked to repeat a meaningful phrase and then a jumble of words, will repeat the meaningful phrase but be unable to remember the unconnected words. An autistic child will have equal difficulty with the phrase and the jumble of words. Normal auditory clues and previous auditory experience are of little help to an autistic child. As an autistic child develops speech he may show articulatory defects and an odd intonation of speech, presumably due to the poor feedback.

In the same way, the child may not comprehend visual stimuli and his obsession with the same small object may be due to his inability to sort out his visual world. The apparent visual avoidance of adults has been found to be a visual avoidance of all external stimuli. An autistic child may look at all objects for a very short time, and then often with peripheral vision.

This difficulty in sorting out the stimuli reaching him from his world appears to be the basis of autism, and it is obvious that varying degrees of the condition exist.

Management

It is possible that with early diagnosis and specific help many cases could be improved. Actually teaching a child understanding of sounds and language from its simplest beginnings, and helping him to appreciate what he sees, might give him the necessary early help.

Simple free play is no good whatsoever. The child will retire into his spinning, twiddling attitude and no progress will be made. He needs a strictly structured environment and programme.

Parents The parents can be helped to structure the environment. The mother can spend time with the child and reward by a smile or a sweet every outgoing sign from him, like a communicative noise or a very simple constructive sign in play, such as putting a toy in a box. In this way the child may find purposeful activities pleasurable and this can lead to toilet training and self dressing.

School Education for these children should start at 3 years of age. Apart from a structured environment, some teachers would praise appropriate actions and use discipline in the form of disapproval for inappropriate actions. It is hoped that making the environment meaningful and consistent at all times may lead to improvement. These methods come under the overall heading of 'behaviour modification'. Different schools use different methods; and at present it is not possible to be sure which method is to be preferred.

Team Liberal staffing of a school or therapy room is needed if these children are to be helped. In fact a 1 : 1 ratio of staff to child is not considered excessive. The disciplines involved can vary. Individual sessions with a speech therapist, starting at the simplest level, may help to build up speech. Often an intelligent untrained helper develops a knack of dealing with these children; and her services may be invaluable.

Elective Mutism

Features of this condition are:
a   Absence of evidence of central or peripheral disturbances of the function of the speech mechanisms
b   Absence of a history of organic illness
c   Complete silence from the child after normal speech and language have been established: either a total silence or silence in specific situations, such as in school.

There is usually an early history of traumatic separations from the parents or a secure substitute figure, or a severe defect in the mother-child relationship. The child has difficulty in making contact with an adult, and appears to retire into his own world. There may be no eye contact and the child does not even use gesture. There is evidence that he can sum up a situation and is using reasoning powers: e.g. a child of $3\frac{1}{2}$ years may show rage when seeing his usual playroom occupied by other children. A child of this type requires prolonged and secure contact with an adult until speech is restored spontaneously in a psychiatrically orientated environment. A social worker must work with the mother and family to correct the tensions and attitudes at home.

REFERENCES

Advice to Parents of Aphasic Children. Moor House School, Oxted, Surrey

ANTHONY A, BOGLE D, INGRAM T T S & MCISAAC M W (1971) *The Edinburgh Articulation Test.* Churchill Livingstone, Edinburgh

BERRY M F & EISENSON J (1956) *Speech Disorders, Principles and Practices of Therapy.* Appleton, New York

BUTLER N, PECKHAM C & SHERIDAN M (1973) 'Speech defects in children aged seven years.' *Brit. med. J.* **1**, 253

CLANCY H, DUGDALE A & RENDLE-SHORT J (1969) The diagnosis of infantile autism. *Dev. Med. Childh. Neurol.* **11**, 4, 432–442

CREAK M (1961) Schizophrenic syndrome in childhood. Progress report of a working party. *Cerebral Palsy Bull.* **3**, 501–504

HASKELL S (1964) *Elective Mutism. A Child who does not Talk.* Heinemann, London

HELLER T (1908) Uber dementia infantilus. *Ztschr. forsch. Behandi Jugenal schivoch-sima* **2**, 17–28

INGRAM T T S (1960) The differential diagnosis of speech disorders in childhood. *Practitioner,* **185**, 188

KANNER L (1943) Autistic disturbances of affective contact. *Nerv. Child.* **2**, 217

LEA J (1968) Language and receptive aphasia. *Spec. Educ.* **57**, 3

LEA J (1970) *The Colour Pattern Scheme. A Method of Remedial Language Teaching.* Moor House School, Oxted, Surrey

MORLEY M E (1962) *Cleft Palate and Speech.* Livingstone, London

MORLEY M E (1968) *The Development and Disorders of Speech in Childhood.* E & S Livingstone, London

RENFREW C & MURPHY K (1964) *The Child who does not Talk. Clinics in Developmental Medicine,* No. 13. Spastics Society & William Heinemann, London

RENFREW C (1972) *Speech Disorders in Children.* Pergamon, Oxford

REYNELL J (1969) A developmental approach to language disorders. *Brit. J. Dis. Comm.* **4**, 1, 33

RUTTER M ed. (1971) *Infantile Autism. Concepts, Characteristics and Treatment.* Study Group 1. Contributors: Kolvin I, Koupernik C, Ornitz E M, Hermelin B, Rutter M, Wing L & Baitak L. Churchill, London

RUTTER M & MARTIN T A [eds.] (1972) *Psychiatric Causes of Language Retardation. The Child with Delayed Speech.* Heinemann, London

WEDELL (1964) *Some Developmental Disorders of Speech in Learning Problem of the Cerebral Palsied.* Spastics Society, London

WORSTER DROUGHT C (1953) Speech disorders of children of school age. *Medical Press* **230**, 149

WORSTER DROUGHT C (1954) Speech disorders in children of school age. *J. RIPH & H* **17**, 190

WORSTER DROUGHT C (1956) Congenital suprabulbar paresis. *J. Laryng.* **70**, 153

WORSTER DROUGHT C (1971) An unusual form of acquired aphasia. *Dev. Med. Childh. Neurol.* **13**, 563

Chapter 15
Congenital Deformities

SPINA BIFIDA CYSTICA
AND ASSOCIATED
CONGENITAL DEFOMITIES

This group of deformities is due to a failure in the development of midline structures. In early uterine life there has been a defect in the fusion of ectoderm, neuroectoderm and mesoderm to form the components of the spinal column—spinal cord and canal, its coverings of dura and arachnoid, the vertebral column and overlying skin and muscle.

Incidence

The incidence varies in different parts of the world and in different parts of one country. It is said to be low in African countries, of the order of 0·32 per 1000 in Japan, and 0·56 per 1000 in Melbourne, Australia. In England the incidence in Liverpool (1965) was 3·5 per 1000 births, excluding anencephalics; and in South Wales (1964) in the region of 10 per 1000, including anencephalics and congenital hydrocephalics. The overall rate in Britain may be 3 per 1000. There is a much lower incidence in the USA.

Aetiology and Genetics

As with many other handicapping conditions the cause is multifactorial. There is a higher than normal incidence of first born children and children of birth orders five or over. There is an increased incidence in the lower social classes, which suggests an environmental factor, and recently blight in potatoes has been suggested as a teratological cause (Renwick 1972).

Family and population studies show that after the birth of a child with a midline deformity of the central nervous system the chances of a further child born with a midline deformity—not necessarily of the same type or of the same severity—is 1 in 12, but the chance of a *surviving* child with a serious deformity is 1 in 25. After two affected children, the chances are 1 in 8.

There are two types of spina bifida cystica.

1   Meningocele

A cystic pedunculated swelling covered by skin or membrane is present along any part of the spinal column, but usually in the lumbosacral region. The skin may be covered by hair or by an angioma. During surgical repair, the cord and nerves are found to lie in the spinal canal and not to be associated with the defect of the vertebral column and overlying skin. There is no lower motor neuron defect, but the defect may however be associated with a malformation of the brain, such as an aqueduct stenosis or Arnold–Chiari malformation. Hydrocephalus may develop after repair of the meningocele.

2   Meningomyelocele

This is a much more serious lesion. The spinal cord and accompanying nerves are involved in the deformity and may be lying exposed or involved in the membranous cover of the cyst. The lesion is usually in the lower thoracic or upper lumbar region, but may be placed more caudally and may involve a large or small area of the vertebral column. There are frequent additional abnormalities of the spinal cord and column which play a part in the total neurological deficit. The spinal canal above the lesion may be enlarged, giving a hydromyelia, or spinal cysts in the canal may occur. Bony or fibrous abnormalities in the spinal column may cause a diastematomyelia. Nearly all children with a myelocele have an Arnold–Chiari malformation. There is a tongue-like projection of the cerebellum which becomes firmly adherent to the medulla, and may extend down through the foramen magnum. Parts of the fourth ventricle may be involved in the abnormality. The downward displacement of cerebral tissue causes displacement and diversion upwards of cranial and cervical nerves, and may account for neurological abnormalities in the upper limb. There may also be a stenosis of the aqueduct of Sylvius.

A child with meningocele or myelocele may show other congenital abnormalities. The list includes:

Vertebral	Sacral agenesis and hemisacra
	Hemivertebrae and deformities of ribs and vertebrae
	Short trunk
Skeletal	Abnormalities of limbs and syndactyly
	Club feet, congenital dislocation of hip and arthrogryposis
Urinary	Megaureters and hydronephrosis
	Vesico-ureteric reflex
	Other renal abnormalities, such as horseshoe kidney
Alimentary	Tracheo-oesophageal fistula, imperforate rectum
Other abnormalities	Cleft palate, congenital heart defect

Early Surgical Management

The child is usually born after an uncomplicated pregnancy and 40 weeks' gestation period. Breech birth occurs in 30% of cases, due to flexed hips and possibly an enlarged head. The defect is noted at birth. At one time it was felt that better results were obtained by immediate operation before dessication or infection of the exposed nerve tissues occurred. It is now felt that, with care to prevent these complications, the operation can be postponed for one to two days, while a decision as to surgery is made.

There is a conflict of opinion as to whether all children should be operated on. If no operation is undertaken, the majority of children die before 5 years of age, and in the past only a very occasional child with an unoperated cyst has survived to attend a school for the physically handicapped. Hide, Parry Williams & Ellis (1972) reported on 99 children who were considered unsuitable for surgery because of complete or nearly complete paralysis of the lower limbs. 92 of the 99 died by one year and only 2 were alive at the end of their four year survey. Some surgeons feel that there is a moral obligation to salvage the lives of all children. Others feel that some selection of cases for surgery must take place.

Lorber (1971) felt that objective data can be used for selection of cases for treatment. He showed that the children who do badly in later life are those with extensive paralysis at birth, a head circumference exceeding the ninetieth percentile, gross hydrocephalus detected by echoencephalography, a gross kyphosis or major associated defects. Other workers would consider two further criteria before embarking on surgery. For them illegitimacy or poor social circumstances would weigh against preserving the life of an affected child, and they would consider it wrong to repair a back and produce a handicapped child when local facilities for medical, rehabilitative and educational care are not available. If surgery is withheld the parents must be given maximum possible support in caring for their child until he dies. Many parents have willingly and devotedly accepted this burden. If the child cannot be sent home from hospital, a suitable ward or home must be provided with nursing care until death occurs.

With the need for early surgery, it is difficult to give the parents, particularly the mother, a full picture of the condition and the likely outcome before she is asked to give written permission for surgery. It is doubtful if it is justifiable to give the parents a choice between surgery and palliative measures only, as they are likely to blame themselves for making the decision, whatever the eventual outcome for the child. It is possibly a paediatrician, in consultation with the family doctor and neurosurgeon, who should decide. A careful assessment of muscle function by a physiotherapist before surgery is of value in making a decision.

Hydrocephalus

After closure of the spinal defect, overt hydrocephalus develops in 70% of cases and enlarged ventricles may be present in nearly 100%. Immediate surgery is needed if the intelligence is to be preserved and it is not safe to wait for a spontaneous arrest. Some surgeons would not operate if the cerebral mantle of cortex is below 15 mm, determined by air ventriculography. Drainage of the cerebrospinal fluid is facilitated by a tube with a no-return valve (Spitz–Holter or Pudenz valve) inserted between the enlarged cerebral ventricles and the jugular vein, superior vena cava or, commonly now, the right auricle. In some children a ventriculoperitoneal shunt is used.

The complications of the operation are infection (ventriculitis) and blockage of the tube, both of which may occur early on but may also occur in later infancy or childhood. As many of these children are living in all parts of the country, and some are attending resident schools for the physically handicapped in rural areas, family doctors and school medical officers must recognise the early signs of these complications and send the child for neurosurgical opinion immediately. Symptoms to watch include irritability, loss of appetite, vomiting, headache, drowsiness, tense fontanelle, enlargement of the head, an appearance of exophthalmos, and a sudden appearance of a bilateral sixth cranial nerve palsy and papilloedema.

To assess whether the system is working, both valves and the intervening connection should be felt behind the ear. If the connection is pressed, it should collapse and slowly refill; failure to collapse or refill should be grounds for referral. The head circumference should be measured regularly. Fifty per cent of children require revision of the tube and valve at least once during infancy and the tube may require to be replaced by a longer tube after a period of growth. Lorber (1972) states that 20% of children die as a result of a complication of the shunt, and he feels that it is an operation that should not be lightly undertaken. Ventriculitis and blockage of the shunt can lead to temporary or permanent blindness, epilepsy or mental retardation from further brain damage.

After surgery to the back, and in the majority of cases the insertion of a shunt because of hydrocephalus, the paediatrician should take over the care of the child.

Paralytic Deformities

The degree of paralysis of the lower limbs varies according to the site of the lesion. Flaccid paralysis of muscles is caused by a lower motor neuron deficit. The paralysis may be complete or there may be minimal function in some muscles. There is a possibility of an upper motor neuron defect caused by a defect in the spinal cord above the level of the back lesion. Some muscles will be functioning normally and the pull of a normal muscle around a joint partially served by flaccid muscles may lead to a joint deformity. Some joint contractures in children with spina bifida are present at birth and resemble arthrogryposis, but may be due to intrauterine muscle imbalance.

There should be a full assessment of the child's muscular function soon after operation. The orthopaedic surgeon, with the help of a physiotherapist, will decide on treatment. The likely clinical state of the muscles according to the level of the lesion is:

Lesion about 3rd lumbar vertebra	Likelihood of total flaccid paraplegia
Lesion between L_4 and S_1	Hip extensors and knee flexors paralysed. Frail feet. Knee extensors, hip flexors and adductors may be retained. There will be bladder and rectal incontinence
Lesion between S_1 and S_3	Hip extensors and knee flexors weak. Paralysed plantar flexion. Weak inversion and eversion of feet. Use of knee extensors, hip flexors and adductors, and dorsiflexors retained. Some use of hip extensors and knee flexors
Below S_3	No paralysis

Management

If the child is to develop normally, emotionally and intellectually, it is important that he achieves an erect position at the normal time or as near to it as possible. He should be mobile and able to explore his environment. He will then develop a knowledge of the world around him in true perspective; and this may go a long way to preventing later learning and perceptual difficulties.

Early physiotherapy is essential. In severe cases the child will need help to attain sitting balance and a triangular floor seat with a tray, similar to the seat used for cerebral palsied children, can enable him to sit and play. There is a danger of flexion contractures of the hips, because the iliopsoas muscle retains its power unapposed; and these children should lie prone on a wedge for a period each day to prevent a flexion deformity. Early surgery, to transplant the psoas muscle for use as an extensor and abductor of the hips, is frequently undertaken.

Later a severely handicapped child will require calipers with a high pelvic brace, to enable him to use his trunk muscles to swing his legs for walking. A Shrewsbury—swivel walker—can give him mobility.

To obtain enjoyable mobility, all severely affected children at the earliest possible age should be given a go-cart or trolley with which they can use their hands to steer themselves around (figure 15.1). One type is the Chailey chariot which in Britain can be obtained from government sources. This makes an enormous difference to the young child's life, and should be considered a 'must' for the paralysed. Later, self-propelled or power-driven wheelchairs should be supplied; whilst at the same time independent walking with long leg braces should be encouraged.

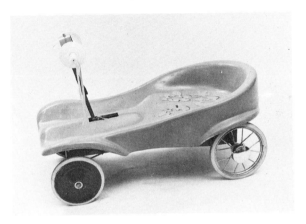

Fig. 15.1 A go-cart which can be used by children with spina bifida, to encourage early mobility and exploration. (By kind permission of the Physiotherapy Department, Royal Victoria Hospital, Melbourne, Australia)

In less severe cases, calipers—either full-length or below knee—made of a light constructional material can be used, with or without crutches or sticks. Surgery may be needed to give a more functional position to the limbs, to correct muscle imbalance, or to correct a dislocated hip or a knee or foot deformity. The 'club feet' type of deformity noted at birth can be corrected by adhesive strapping at first, with close supervision of the skin.

The child should learn to put on his own calipers.

Spinal Defects

Surgery to ameliorate spinal defects may be undertaken during childhood. In severe cases of total paralysis, the removal of one or two vertebrae may correct a disfiguring kyphus over which a skin ulcer can easily develop.

Skin Ulceration

Because of the nerve damage, there will be a sensory loss of the lower limbs with a distribution directly associated with the level of the cord lesion. In sacral lesions without motor involvement there is likely to be anaesthesia around the sacral area, genitalia and anus. In severe cases there may be a total sensory loss from the waist downwards. There is a constant danger of skin ulceration. The child will not notice burning from being too near a fire, or the rubbing of an ill-fitting caliper. Ulceration can occur at all the pressure points. The spinal kyphus is a vulnerable area and the skin of the buttocks which is sodden with urine is at particular risk. Parents of children with spina bifida, and later the child himself, must inspect all the skin areas twice a day to notice any early signs of redness or excoriation. The child should have a mirror placed low in the bathroom or in the toilet area of a special school to see all his skin area. Ulceration, if it does occur, is particularly difficult to heal, due to the lack of innervation and trophic changes in the skin. Skin-grafting may be needed to cure severe ulceration but is not always successful.

Fractures

Due to absence of sensation, lower limb fractures can occur and not be detected for some time, and osteoporosis of the bones increases the hazard. Exuberant callus formation may draw attention to the underlying fracture. James (1970) found an incidence of 18% of cases who had a fracture. Minimal injury may cause a fracture in an atrophic bone, and fractures should be looked for in any child who appears ill.

Urinary Tract Involvement

Due to the spinal cord lesion, virtually all children with this condition are likely to be incontinent of urine, even if the lower limb muscle involvement is minimal. There is the added complication of congenital urinary tract abnormalities in about 20% of cases. An intravenous pyelogram (IVP) should be done soon after birth. Some paediatricians would insist on an IVP before deciding on surgical closure of the myelomeningocele, and would not advise operation on a child with an abnormal urinary tract.

The urinary complications likely to develop are:

Infection

Damage to kidneys from ureteric reflux and infection

Incontinence

Urinary Infection has been found to occur in 25% of cases at 6 months and 50% of cases at 18 months. By 5 years of age 30% of children have a chronic infection which cannot be eradicated; and by 8 years of age 90% of children have had a urinary infection. Most workers would suggest that the urine should be examined at regular intervals. It can be tested by examining the specimen for pus and organisms under a high power microscope at a regular clinic. Urine specimens can be sent routinely for full investigation to a laboratory. The parents can be given a 'uricult' set to test the urine at home and report to the doctor when bacterial growth is present, and if the parents are intelligent the last method may be preferable.

Infection should be treated by antibiotics, but prolonged use may not prevent recurrent infection. Possibly the treatment should be given when an infection is present and be brief and effective. Prophylactically the child should be encouraged to drink frequently. A local antibiotic cream such as tetracycline cream should be applied to the genitals to prevent urinary infection.

Bladder Dysfunction The bladder may be neurologically impaired in one of two ways. It may be flaccid with urinary incontinence and sometimes dribbling of urine, and infection may occur from the inability to empty the bladder completely. A totally flaccid bladder can be emptied by repeated expression. The child lies on his back; a warm hand is placed below the umbilicus and pressure is placed on the bladder by a downward and backward movement. This can be done from 6 months of age onwards after every meal, and in an occasional case this method of urinary control is totally satisfactory and the child remains dry and free from infection.

Alternatively there may be bladder-neck obstruction from neurologically determined transurethral spasm. This leads to retention of urine, infection and trabeculation of the bladder, ureteric reflux and kidney damage. Surgical transurethral resection of the bladder neck may be required. Children with urethral obstruction should not be treated with bladder expression, as this will increase the likelihood of ureteric reflux.

To make an early diagnosis of bladder function, the onset of ureteric reflux, and the development of hydroureter, hydronephrosis or renal stones, there should be routine investigations at regular intervals. A micturating cystogram can be undertaken at 2 years of age. An intravenous pyelogram should be done as a routine at 6 months, 2 years, 4 years and 6 years of age. Regular biochemical studies of renal function and measurements of blood pressure should take place, even if the child is living at a long distance from a hospital.

Gross kidney damage can occur in mildly affected children and is a common cause of death, and all children should be under the constant care of a urologist, with referral to a urogenital surgeon.

Urinary Incontinence In all but a small proportion of children with spina bifida, urinary incontinence becomes a major problem. For some children, urinary diversion must be undertaken. The indications for the operation are:
Uncontrolled infection
Increasing upper urinary tract damage
Incontinence over the age of 5 years in a girl

The operation is a cutaneous ureterostomy, in which both ureters are brought to the abdominal surface, or an ileum or sigmoid loop ureostomy. In these last two operations, the ureters are diverted into an isolated portion of gut, which is brought to the surface to form a protuberant opening or spout from which the urine drains. The spout should protrude for at least an inch so that a bag can be worn without any leaking of urine. It should be placed anteriorly on the abdominal wall so that the child can later be independent in the use of an appliance.

The child wears a close-fitting belt and a polythene collecting bag for the urine. The apparatus consists of a flange, a two-sided sticky patch, a bag, a metal ring and a supporting belt. The skin is treated with friars' balsam or alcohol, and the flange and sticky patch are removed only once a week. The bag is fitted on to a metal ring which is fitted to the flange, and is emptied regularly. The use of this apparatus by many children can be very successful. While using it, the child can lead a normal life and can take part in swimming and other activities. The non-functioning bladder may become infected and a persistent purulent discharge per urethra may cause discomfort.

For boys, a urinal or penile bag attached to an abdominal belt can be successfully used and can keep the child dry and clean. He should use a new polythene bag daily to prevent infection.

In cases of persistent infection due to ureteric reflux in boys, a diversionary operation similar to the operation for girls may be a lifesaving measure.

Faecal Incontinence

An intelligent child who has received no training may remain totally incontinent of faeces. Others may have faecal impaction and overflow incontinence.

Faecal continence can be obtained. Regular toileting half an hour after the evening meal, with or without the use of a purgative such as Dulcodos tablets or Senokot syrup, may achieve a normal bowel action daily. Sometimes the use of suppositories or microenemata is necessary, or a bland drug such as Isogel can be given to add bulk to the faeces. If urinary continence is obtained by a diversionary operation, the child has more incentive to be bowel-trained. Recently a method called "sacral beating" has been introduced from Hungary. A firm rhythmic beat on the sacrum can induce bowel and urinary flow. A child can learn to use this stimulus independently.

In cases of a lax and patulous anus, surgical reconstruction to form a functioning anus by using the gracilis muscle has been successful.

Early menstruation, sometimes around 7 years of age, may occur in girls due to internal hydrocephalus and hypothalamic involvement.

Early Training

The child with spina bifida is one with several handicaps, all of which require medical treatment, and in many cases surgery. The mother has to attend several consultant clinics and centres for therapy. These frequent attendances may impose an impossible burden on her if she has other young children to care for. Ideally a polyclinic should be set up for these children, so that all routine consultant attendances can be fitted in on the same day and in the same location.

Due either to lack of early mobility and play or to neurological involvement of the upper limbs, many of these children have little skill in the use of their hands. The child may remain unduly dependent on his mother for feeding and dressing. He may show the spatial visuomotor and perceptual difficulties that have been observed in children with brain damage or with cerebral palsy. At the same time these children may develop speech early and be 'chatterers', but may be using words and language ahead of their understanding. The language used may have little meaning for the child and be purely repetitive or attention-seeking, and in this way he may be similar to a blind child. This condition has been called the 'cocktail' syndrome—the chatter resembling that at a cocktail party.

Some of these difficulties may be due to cerebral abnormalities or pathology, but it is felt that with some children the condition has been caused by the early lack of attaining the erect posture, of becoming mobile and of having opportunities to play. This aspect of the child's training should be supervised from the earliest months, and specific advice on play, stimulation and mobility should be given to the mother.

Education

Nursery school education should be considered a 'must' for these handicapped children. With extra help in the classroom, the majority should fit into normal schools at 5 years. The most severe problem is incontinence. In some areas the mother will collect the child from school in the lunch hour to attend to his toilet needs. If several of these children in one area could attend the same school, the addition of a nurse to the staffing establishment would mean that toileting, calipers and skin ulceration problems could be adequately dealt with while the child receives a normal education. Later on it is hoped that all but the most severely handicapped children will be independent for everyday needs. Swimming should be encouraged, to develop strong shoulder muscles able to cope with lower limb appliances. Obesity may occur due to immobility, and the child's diet should be carefully watched.

Mental Retardation

There will be a small minority of these children who will be mentally retarded due to additional cerebral abnormality, severe hydrocephalus or cerebral damage caused by ventriculitis. Some of these children will be epileptic, and Lorber (1972) reported 13 epileptic children among 103 survivors. A few will be blind due to the cerebral complications. These very handicapped children will need purpose-planned provision.

Outcome

A follow-up of all treated cases of myelomeningocele in Sheffield (Lorber 1972) showed that no survivor was without a physical defect. In many schools for the physically handicapped, the number of children with this condition at present exceeds that of cerebral palsy cases.

OTHER CONGENITAL ABNORMALITIES AFFECTING MOBILITY

A child may be born with absent or deformed limbs, or limbs which function abnormally. The various types are described below.

Dysmelia

The descriptive terms used for different abnormalities are:

Amelia   Complete absence of arm or leg.

Phocomelia   Complete absence of all long bones of the limbs (humerus, radius, ulna, femur, tibia and fibula). A malformed hand or foot only is present.

Axial ectromelia   Disturbance of development involving the humerus, radius and radial ray of the hand, or the femur, tibia and tibial ray of the foot.

Proximal ectromelia   Found in lower limb only. The proximal part of the femur only is involved.

Distal ectromelia   Malformations involving either the radius and radial ray of the hand or the tibia and tibial ray of the foot.

Perimelia   Part of a limb is totally missing, with normal anatomy proximal to the absence.

At the present time in Britain and many European countries, the majority of children with dysmelia, apart from perimelia, were born between 1959 and 1962. Taking of the drug thalidomide between the twenty-eight and forty-second day of pregnancy has been blamed. In some cases the history of medication is indefinite, but the similarity of the cases suggests a similar aetiology. Only one tablet may have been taken. Apart from this epidemic, only occasional cases occur and in any large area a case is likely to be seen only once in a few years. Goya made a drawing of an affected child titled 'A Mother revealing her Deformed Child'.

Different degrees of dysmelia are seen. The arms alone may be affected, with normal legs; or all four limbs may be involved. The phocomelic arms may be represented by a few fingers attached to the shoulder or to a shortened limb. The humerus, which may be dislocated at the shoulder joint, and the elbow joint, radius and ulna, if present, may be very abnormal. The thumb is often absent, and even in cases where five fingers are present, it may be that none can be opposed to the other. Comparable deformities occur in the lower limbs.

There may be other congenital abnormalities present. The list includes:

Capillary naevi on the face

Anophthalmia, microphthalmia. Misplaced or single eye. Blindness

Absence of ear. Abnormal alignment or absence of ossicles. Deafness

Abnormalities of gastrointestinal tract—stenosis or atresia of oesophagus, duodenum or anus

Maldevelopment of heart or lungs

Anomalies of renal tract

Perimelia

These cases are called intrauterine amputations and may be due to restricting amniotic bands cutting off blood supply to the limbs during intrauterine life. Upper limb defects are five times commoner than lower limb defects. In some cases there is evidence of dominant or recessive inheritance of the condition.

Malformations of Hands or Feet

Congenital anomalies include absent thumbs, fingers or toes, syndactyly and polydactyly. Some cases need surgery, but the condition need not cause a major physical handicap and children can live a normal life with these defects.

Arthrogryposis Multiplex Congenita

In children born with this condition abnormalities in several joints are noted at birth. Various joints may be involved, but usually the large joints of the arms and legs are ankylosed in extension. The arms are rotated inwards and the hands and wrists sharply flexed. The thighs are rotated outwards with slight flexion of the hips, extended knees, and feet in the equinovarus position. There is marked rigidity and immobility of the affected joints, and an absence or maldevelopment of muscles round the joints. Some children have a small recessed chin, and the range of movement of the jaw is limited. The cause of the condition may be multifactorial, hereditary, intrauterine or environmental.

The actual nature of the deformities is difficult to determine. It may be due to an intrauterine lesion of upper motor neurons or lower motor neurons, or maldevelopment of muscles or joints.

Congenital Dislocation of Hip, Club Feet, Syndactyly

Congenital deformities of this type can be corrected early and should not prevent a child leading a normal life. Additional handicaps such as mental retardation may be present, and all these children should be assessed to eliminate the possibility of other handicapping defects.

Management

As these grosser abnormalities are comparatively rare, it is unlikely that personnel working in a medium-sized conurbation will have had experience of these handicaps. Expert opinion of the best methods to help a child will have to be obtained from an established centre where specialised knowledge is available. It may be advantageous to organise a visit for the handicapped child, his parents and the therapist involved, to obtain advice on overall management; and it may be preferable if the mother and child can be resident at the centre while appliances are fitted and training in their use is given.

Marquardt (1962) made the following points about treatment (figure 15.2):

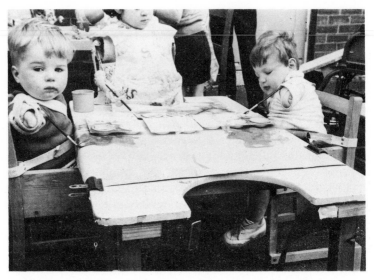

Fig. 15.2 Two children with dysmelia, using appliances which will encourage early play and manual skills.

a   The parents must be given early information about treatment and future outlook.

b   The child should grow up in the family.

c   Early physiotherapy and occupational therapy should be given.

d   The mother is the child's best therapist.

e   The clothes must be altered so that the deformed hands, fingers and feet may touch and grasp without hindrance.

f   In the case of absent arms, the baby must have an opportunity to watch his feet and play with them. The bed covers should be taken off during the day.

g   Small hands and digits coming directly from the shoulders must be incited to touch and grasp. They will be needed later to control prostheses.

h   In the absence of all four limbs, the child must be encouraged to use his mouth.

i   The armless child should lie prone on a wooden board to strengthen his back.

j   In armless babies, feet and toes must be trained.

k   Surgical corrections of deformities should be conducted only from the aspect of function.

l   Above average flexibility of hips is necessary if the child is to use his lower limbs for dressing and undressing.

m   A helmet must be used with an armless baby to protect his head if he falls.

n   A child who can eat and play with his deformed hands does not need a prosthesis.

Children with *upper limb deformities* must have an early sense of body symmetry to prevent scoliosis and to give a normal body image. A child with a one arm defect should be fitted from babyhood with a rounded stump so that he gets a sensation through his defective limb and learns early the value of using both arms. At about 1 year of age a simple prosthesis, such as a flexible cuff, can be fitted. A spoon, paintbrush or pencil can be fitted between the cuff and the stump, which the child will learn to use. In cases of ectromelia, the defective arm may grow, and later the disproportion between arm, head and trunk may be reduced. The child may then be able to use a long spoon or pencil held in his malformed fingers.

At about 2 years of age a child can be fitted with a conventional upper limb prosthesis with hinged joints and a hook or artificial hand attached. Tuition must be given in its use. At 4–5 years children with weak muscles, or minimal muscular control at the shoulder or elbow joint, can be fitted with a pneumatic prosthesis, which involves the use of carbon dioxide in containers worn around the body, and which gives additional power to the artificial limb by a valve action.

The value and purpose of the prosthesis must be kept under review. It is found that many children discard them later and prefer to make their own adjustment. This often involves using the feet for activities such as feeding, writing, typing and other skills. If the child is adept in using his feet, it seems doubtful that this should be discouraged. The general public nowadays willingly accept this abnormality. A man with no arms has been seen to open the car door for a lady with his feet, and this type of use is socially entirely acceptable.

A child with *defective lower limbs* should achieve an erect posture and an ability to move and explore at the correct developmental age. Children with lower limb phocomelia can be fitted into a type of flowerpot prosthesis. Movements can be obtained by trunk rotation. More detailed prosthesis can be fitted later with a pelvic brace. The child may use the prosthesis in the physiotherapy department more efficiently and conscientiously than he does at home or school. If he has developed skills of independence in the centre, it must be ascertained that he is also using this new-found independence at home and school, and is not being made unnecessarily dependent on others.

Surgery

The surgeon considering operative interference in the child's deformity must have an opinion from an occupational therapist or physiotherapist, or, in their absence, a very detailed description of the child's abilities from the parents. In the club feet deformity in arthrogryposis, surgery is needed to obtain stable flat feet on which the child can walk. In upper limb deformities, he may achieve many tasks by the combined use of both arms. With two extended arms with minimal elbow flexion he may be able to pick things up and hold a pen to write. To give him one flexed and one straight arm may reduce these skills, and surgery of this type needs careful consideration. If a child is using his feet, surgical straightening of a flexed hip may adversely affect his independence. It is open to question whether the child would not lead a happier life in a wheelchair, with flexed hips, able to use his feet. In early surgery every particle of skin on extra digits and other parts must be retained, as it may be useful later for cosmetic surgery.

Schools

These children need all the normal experiences of play, and early attendance at a nursery school is desirable. If there are no serious additional handicaps likely to interfere with education, the child should attend a normal school. It is hoped that enlightened education authorities will provide the school with an additional pair of hands to help the integration of the child into normal school life. It has been said that normal children of 5 years are curious about these abnormal children but unembarrassed and unimpressed by them, and will accept and help them in a straightforward manner.

Congenital Cardiac and Other Defects

There are a group of children with chronic illness due to a developmental abnormality, who come under the overall heading of handicapped children. A description of the medical condition is more appropriately dealt with in textbooks of general paediatrics. Due to modern therapeutic techniques the number requiring special schooling has been dramatically reduced.

Cardiac Defects

The majority of congenital cardiac defects are amenable to corrective surgery, which means that the child with this type of defect can lead an active life at ordinary school with a few defined precautions. The parents must be encouraged to allow the child as normal a life as possible, both before and after surgery; and school medical officers should be orientated to the new outlook for children with congenital heart defects. Only children with inoperable conditions such as tricuspid atresia, single ventricle, and pulmonary artery atresia with intact ventricular wall may need special school placement; and the majority of these die early.

There are unfortunately children who have undergone cardiac surgery in schools for the physically handicapped who should be attending their neighbourhood schools.

There are a minority of children who have additional handicaps, and children with cardiac abnormalities should have a general paediatric assessment. Gardner (1969) has shown that 36% have a visual refractive error (24% myopic and 12% hypermetropic). The condition may be associated with other congenital defects such as harelip, cleft palate, submucous cleft, scoliosis and limb abnormalities. It is well known that 8%–10% of children with Down's syndrome have cardiac defects; and a cardiac defect may occur in other children with severe mental retardation. These children should have cardiac surgery if appropriate. In 1958 it was found that in one hospital for 700 mentally subnormal patients 70 (10%) had a congenital heart defect. The majority, but not all, had Down's syndrome.

Cystic Fibrosis

The majority of children with cystic fibrosis will require special schooling. They are undersized, lacking in general physical stamina, have repeated bronchial infections and require daily postural drainage by a physiotherapist. Possibly the most suitable school for them would be a school designated as a 'School for Delicate Children' (see chapter 17).

REFERENCES

D'AVIGNON M, HELLGREN K, JUHLIN M & ATTERBACH B (1967) Diagnostic and habilitation problems of thalidomide traumatized children with multiple handicaps. *Dev. Med. Childh. Neurol.* **9**, 6

DEPARTMENT OF HEALTH AND SOCIAL SECURITY (1973) *Care of the Child with Spina Bifida.* HMSO, London

ELLISON & NASH D F (1969) Urinary problems of spina bifida. *Dev. Med. Childh. Neurol.* **11**, 1, 105

FIELD A (1970) *The Challenge of Spina Bifida.* Heinemann, London

FORSYTHE W I & KINLEY J G (1970) Bowel control of children with spina bifida. *Dev. Med. Childh. Neurol.* **12**, 1, 27

HAUSEN E (1968) Arthrogryposis multiplex congenita. *Dev. Med. Childh. Neurol.* **10**, 1, 109

HIDE D W, PARRY WILLIAMS H & ELLIS H L (1972) The outlook for the child with a meningocele for whom early surgery was considered inadvisable. *Dev. Med. Childh. Neurol* **14**, 3, 309

LAURENCE K M & TEW B J (1971) Natural history of spina bifida and cranium bifida. *Arch. Dis. Childh.* **46**, 127

LORBER J (1971) Results of treatment of myelomeningocele. *Dev. Med. Childh. Neurol.* **13**, 279

LORBER J (1972) *Your Child with Spina Bifida.* Association for Spina Bifida and Hydrocephalus, London

LORBER J (1972) Spina bifida results of treatment of 270 consecutive cases. *Arch. Dis. Childh.* **47**, 256, 854

MARQUARDT E (1962) *Information on Measures for Habilitation of Children with Dysmelia.* Deutsche Vereingure fur die Rehabilitation Behinderter, Heidelberg

NIXON (1972) *Proc. Roy. Soc. Med.*—not yet published

NORMAN A P ed. (1968) *Congenital Abnormalities in Infancy.* Blackwell, Oxford

RENWICK J H (1972) Potato babies. *Lancet*, **2**, 336

ROBERTSON E S (1971) *Follow-up Study into the Functional Abilities at Home and at School of Multiple Limb Deficient Children.* Children's Prosthetic Unit, Queen Mary's Hospital, Roehampton

SHARRARD W(1971) Arthrogryposis multiplex congenital, pp. 454–461. In *Paediatric Orthopaedics and Fractures.* Blackwell, Oxford

SHARRARD W (1971) Congenital and developmental abnormalities of the neuraxis, pp. 596–691. In *Paediatric Orthopaedics and Fractures.* Blackwell, Oxford

SMITH E D (1965) *Spina Bifida and the Total Care of Myelomeningocele.* C C Thomas, Illinois

SYMPOSIUM (1965) *Spina Bifida.* National Fund for Research into Crippling Diseases, London

STEPHEN E (1963) Intelligence levels and educational status of children with meningomyelocele. *Dev. Med. Childh. Neurol.* **5**, 572

Studies in hydrocephalus and spina bifida (1968) *Dev. Med. Childh. Neurol. Supplement 15.* Heinemann, London

Studies in hydrocephalus and spina bifida (1970) *Dev. Med. Childh. Neurol. Supplement 22.* Heinemann, London

Studies in hydrocephalus and spina bifida (1971) *Dev. Med. Childh. Neurol. Supplement 25.* Heinemann, London

Studies in hydrocephalus and spina bifida (1973) *Dev. Med. Childh. Neurol. Supplement 29.* Heinemann, London

SWISHER L P & PINSKER E J (1971) The language characteristics of hyperverbal hydrocephalic children. *Dev. Med. Childh. Neurol.* **13**, 6, 746

WALKER J H, THOMAS M & RUSSELL I T (1971) Spina bifida and the parents. *Dev. Med. Childh. Neurol.* **13**, 4, 462

Chapter 16
The Child who Becomes Handicapped

A normal, active, intelligent child may become permanently physically handicapped in childhood from a variety of causes. It appears justifiable to include all these conditions in one chapter, as a child who slowly deteriorates physically poses difficulties in diagnosis and school placement to the school medical officer, family doctor or paediatrician. The child's difficulties may be noted first by the parents or class teachers. Until a firm diagnosis is made, he may suffer very seriously from a lack of appreciation of his difficulties.

Visually Handicapped Child

The more common conditions causing gradual and permanent disability are:

Trauma to the eye

Tumour involving the eye and orbit

Congenital syphilis and other infection

Genetically determined deteriorating eye conditions, such as retinitis pigmentosa and tapetoretinal degeneration

Intracranial tumour involving the optic chiasma, optic nerves and pathways

Cerebral trauma involving the optic pathways or occipital cortex

These conditions have been dealt with in chapter 5. It must be emphasised that in school the first sign of incipient eye disease may be the development of a squint.

Hearing Impaired Child

The child may become deaf from comparable conditions involving the middle and inner ear and the auditory pathways. These conditions have been dealt with in chapter 3.

Epileptic Child

A child may develop epilepsy in childhood, and every case should be fully investigated. The condition may be associated with many of the handicapping conditions mentioned in this book. Isolated idiopathic epilepsy should not be considered a handicapping condition during school life. If the child conscientiously takes medication and leads a comparatively well-organised and emotionally secure life, the incidence of fits should not prevent him from leading a normal life and attending normal school. His classmates are usually helpful and sympathetic and undisturbed by the occasional fits. Problems unfortunately arise when he leaves school and tries to obtain employment and lodging. Where home circumstances are unfavourable, and in the occasional case where the fits are not controlled, admission to a special school for epileptics may be necessary. In the majority of cases, a poorly controlled epileptic admitted to one of these schools becomes free from fits during term time.

Neurological Deterioration

Acute illness, such as meningitis or encephalitis, particularly after measles, may leave a hitherto normal child permanently damaged neurologically and mentally. Gradual deterioration may be due to a subacute encephalitis or one of the genetically determined conditions described under mental retardation in chapter 11. Lead encephalopathy is an occasional cause.

Disorders of Mobility

Conditions causing disorders of mobility are:

Cortical Brain Damage

Cerebral tumour
Cerebrovascular abnormalities
Cerebral anoxia—cardiac arrest
Head injuries and battered baby syndrome

These last three conditions may lead to unilateral or bilateral hemiplegia.

Upper Motor Neuron Disease

Friedreich's ataxia
Ataxia telangiectasia
Dystonia musculorum deformans

Lower Motor Neuron Disease

Spinal cord trauma
Progressive spinal muscular atrophy—the childhood form of
   Werdnig–Hoffmann's disease
Anterior poliomyelitis

Diseases of Peripheral Nerves

Various forms of polyneuritis

Diseases of Motor End Plate

Myasthenia gravis

Myopathies (muscle fibre disease)

Muscular dystrophy
Dystrophia myotonica
Polymyositis

Diseases of Joints

Rheumatoid arthritis—Still's disease

Diseases of Bone

Osteogenesis imperfecta—fragilitas ossium

In many of these cases, almost imperceptible deterioration in movement takes place and the child on examination may present as a 'clumsy' child. With the parents' permission, it is important to find out from the class teacher whether she can say from memory if the child has always been incoordinated, or if there has been a slow deterioration. Electromyography, muscle biopsy, estimations of nerve conduction and specific enzyme estimations may be needed to establish the diagnosis.

The commoner conditions occurring in schoolchildren are described below.

Head Injuries

The majority of all head injuries in children fall into two categories. Before the age of 3 years the largest number occur in the home and are due to accidental falls or baby battering, for which the terms child abuse or non-accidental injury are also used. After the age of 3 years accidents are more likely to occur outside the home, mainly due to injuries when the child is either riding a bicycle, crossing a road or climbing adventurously. There is a peak of incidence at 9 years of age. Very few accidents occur at school. Accidents occurring in early and late adolescence have some relationship to periods of stress or maladjustment, and it is not uncommon for children to have a serious accident before an examination. There has been a six-fold increase in head injuries in children during the last twenty years.

Battered Baby

Permanent brain damage may occur as a result of baby battering in infancy; and this condition must be considered if there is evidence of bruising on parts of the body as well as the head. Often there is evidence of present and past fractures. It can occur in all social classes, and poor housing conditions, loneliness and unhappiness in the parents may be a cause. Often the parents themselves were exposed to physical punishment and violence as children. These families, with a child that they have damaged themselves, need careful handling. If the child is only bruised and no sequelae are likely, support from a social worker may prevent a further occurrence. If the battering has resulted in permanent brain damage it is questionable that the child should be returned to the parents. The overriding need is to help the damaged child with retraining.

If the baby remains with his parents, therapists, teachers and social workers must support and befriend them at all times. It is no help to the parents to feel continuously condemned by those around them; and it may be better to carry on with therapy and parent help, and not mention the incident that caused the accident. The parents may later find themselves able to talk about it. At the same time, therapists must watch for any evidence of further injury.

Accidents Causing Brain Injury

In the majority of cases of head injury, even involving a penetrating injury or a period of unconsciousness, there are no sequelae and the child makes a perfect recovery. A minority are left with permanent damage, cortical blindness due to damage to the occipital lobe, unilateral or bilateral hemiplegia, or a cortical speech defect. In one survey (Craft 1973) 4 out of 200 cases had a permanent neurological defect. However, children are more likely to show an overall deterioration of cortical function, whereas adults with a similar injury are more likely to have a focal lesion. A pulsating bony skull defect should be closed by a bone graft, or the child may be restricted in his school activities.

After the child has recovered from the acute sequelae of the accident, he should have a full assessment and come under the care of a paediatrician. There may be a motor defect, a field of vision defect or astereognosis in the affected limb. An EEG should be performed to exclude the possibility of future epilepsy.

The child should be stimulated as soon as he recovers consciousness, and a teacher in a hospital ward can help him in his progress back to normality. The teacher may have to take the severely damaged child through the early learning of shapes and colours and of motor skills by the use of sand, water and paint. The child may lose all verbal skills, both receptive and executive; and early retraining must be undertaken.

Before he returns to school, the child should see a psychologist. He may have learning difficulties, a visuomotor disorder, a body image defect or a defect of auditory and immediate memory. He may still have the speech which he had before the accident but without the understanding. There should be a report on the child before the accident from the class teacher, as a proportion of children who have serious accidents were hyperactive and distractible or educationally subnormal children. It has been found that the child's poor performance after an accident is no different from his performance before the accident.

He should return to school as soon as possible. Depression, frustration and behaviour disorders can develop, and the impetus to overcome handicaps may be lost. After a head injury the child may show uninhibited behaviour, or he may have periods of 'switching off'. Some children develop episodic violent behaviour and others become euphoric. Young adolescent boys may become particularly difficult in the post-traumatic phase. Nurses have found that abnormally aggressive sexual advances can make it difficult to manage the child in an all female ward. As soon as possible the boy should be supervised by men—male nurses and schoolmasters.

If the speech centre has been damaged, frequent speech therapy should be arranged immediately. An occupational therapist may help the child to regain his skills of self-care, dressing himself and attending to toilet needs. He may need special help in relearning skills such as riding a bicycle.

As there is a danger of permanent epilepsy, anticonvulsant medication, even if fits are not occurring, may be given for two years. It is felt that phenobarbitone is not the correct drug as it is liable to increase hyperactive behaviour.

The parents need support after the accident, particularly if they feel that they are in any way to blame for it. Many symptoms shown by children after head injuries, such as headaches, are emotional in origin and can be eliminated by sensible handling.

Friedreich's Ataxia

This condition is inherited as an autosomal recessive gene. Clumsiness at games and unsteadiness are the first symptoms. The ataxia is worse in darkness or when the eyes are closed. The first deformity noticed is often a pes cavus, but later the muscle reflexes may be absent and the vibration and position sense impaired, due to involvement of the posterior columns. Muscle atrophy increases and skeletal deformities develop as the ventral columns are involved. There is later involvement of the heart muscle. Diabetes and optic atrophy may develop. The child becomes chairbound during adolescence, and death occurs between 20 and 50 years.

Ataxia Telangiectasia

Ataxia telangiectasia is an autosomal recessive disease. There is increasing cerebellar ataxia during childhood. Telangiectasiae appear on the skin and in the conjunctivae between 4 and 6 years. Muscular weakness and deterioration in intelligence are noticed. These children are particularly liable to respiratory infections, as there is a lack of IgA gamma globulin in about two-thirds of the cases. Pathologically there is atrophy of the cerebellum and the thymus. Death occurs in adolescence.

Dystonia Musculorum Deformans (Torsion Spasm)

This condition may be an autosomal dominant condition or it may arise unexpectedly in families due to an autosomal recessive gene. The onset is before puberty and starts with slow involuntary twitching of the limb and inward turning of the feet. The involuntary movements eventually involve the whole body. The face grimaces and the child has difficulty with feeding. He gradually deteriorates. Convulsions do not occur and the intelligence remains unchanged. Chlordiazepoxide, diazepam and artane have been useful as muscle relaxants. Neurosurgical procedures to the basal ganglia have been helpful.

Anterior Poliomyelitis

Disability is caused by a viral infection which attacks the large nerve cells of the lower motor neurons in the spinal cord and the medulla oblongata. After the acute illness affected children show random and asymmetric weakness and wasting of muscles. The condition is non-progressive and treatment to increase residual function should start as soon as the acute illness is over and should continue for several years.

A neurologist or physiotherapist should assess the exact extent of the muscle involvement. There may be surviving nerve cells to innervate muscle fibres; and in any muscle there may be some healthy muscle fibres which can hypertrophy and increase in strength with active training and physiotherapy. Splints and calipers, or a spinal brace, can be used to support weak muscles and prevent overaction of stronger opposing muscles. The affected muscles do not grow, and in consequence the bones also do not grow and become shortened and atrophied. Muscle imbalance may cause deformities such as kyphoscoliosis. Orthopaedic procedures may strengthen movement by transferring the insertion of healthy muscle tendons to augment a weaker movement.

The value of treatment and help has been shown by a nurse and physiotherapist team in Kenya. They have visited isolated villages and treated Africans with longstanding after effects of anterior polio-myelitis. Crutches, sticks, calipers, braces and raised boots have been supplied (figure 16.1). By the use of serial plasters, deformities such as equinus have been partially corrected; and afterwards the patient has been able to wear a raised boot and achieve independent walking.

Cases are rare in schoolchildren in many parts of the world today, due to intensive immunisation campaigns in the early months of life.

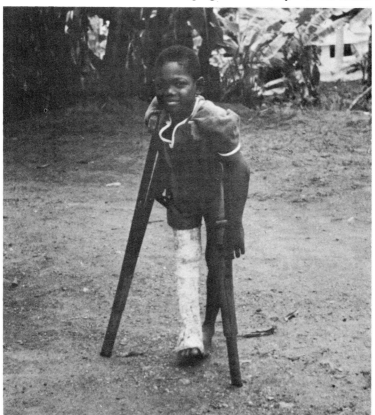

Fig. 16.1 A boy suffering from poliomyelitis who is being treated by simple remedial plasters and being helped to walk with crutches.

Myasthenia Gravis

This condition may arise spontaneously in a family or be inherited as an autosomal recessive. The defect is at the neuromuscular junction and the predominant sympton is undue fatiguability of skeletal muscles. The neuromuscular block can be demonstrated by showing the decrease in muscle response to repeated electric stimulation.

The children are normally active in the morning but become increasingly disabled as the day progresses. Typically there is a ptosis of the eyelids. A subcutaneous injection of neostigmine (0·1 to 1·5 mg) restores muscle power in 5 to 10 minutes and the effect lasts half an hour to 2 hours. This test is diagnostic.

The treatment is by drugs with an anticholinesterase effect, such as tensilon or neostigmine, and can be given by mouth. Thymectomy is performed in severe cases.

The juvenile form may start in early childhood or later and there may be remissions and exacerbations.

Muscular Dystrophy

In this condition there is degeneration of muscle fibres, progressing to nearly total incapacity and death from respiratory failure in late adolescence. The incidence is approximately 1 per 6000 schoolchildren. There are several different conditions with differing modes of inheritance and varying outcomes.

Duchenne type (pseudohypertrophic)   See below.

Becker type   Inherited as sex-linked recessive but milder than Duchenne type. There is a milder form which occurs in girls.

Limb girdle type   Inherited as autosomal recessive affecting the shoulder and pelvic girdles and proximal muscles.

Facio scapulo humeral type   Inherited as autosomal dominant.

Ocular and oculopharyngeal types occur rarely.

Duchenne Type

This form of muscular dystrophy is a sex-linked dominant condition which is passed on by a female carrier to an average of one in two of her male offspring. There is a biochemical enzyme defect in children who have the disease and in females who are the carriers. The serum creatine kinase is increased often to a hundred times above normal in affected boys; and about half this rate in 50% of carrier females. There is also a more specific rise in the level of lactic dehydrogenase isoenzyme 2. The diagnosis can be confirmed without doubt by these tests and also by muscle biopsy. Confirmed female carriers must be told that if they have male children 1 in 2 is likely to be affected, and if they have female children 1 in 2 is likely to be a carrier.

There is a rarer recessive form, which can occur in children of either sex. The disease in one-third of cases is a new mutation.

Children with muscular dystrophy have often caused some concern from babyhood. The child may be late in walking and may never learn to climb stairs. Parents may have remarked on poor balance and frequent falls.

It is soon noticed that there is a weakness of muscles around the pelvic girdle. Abduction of the thighs is weak, giving an early false suggestion of tightness of the adductors. The abdominal and back muscles may be weak, so that the child has difficulty getting up from the floor. He typically gets up by supporting his hands on his legs and gradually crawls up himself. The child early starts to walk on his toes, and this again may suggest a diagnosis of spastic paraplegia. However the tightness of the heel cords appears to be a shortening rather than a spasticity. The calf muscles, although weak, become hypertrophied, giving the typical Hercules appearance, which misleads parents about the muscle weakness. Gradually contractures develop around the hips, knees and ankles. Kyphoscoliosis and weakness of the shoulder and arm muscles occur and the child becomes chairbound at about the age of 10 years. Power in the intrinsic muscles of the hands is usually retained. Movement of the limbs and the deformed joints may be painful.

There is no specific treatment, but much can be done to help the child and consequently make the family situation happier. Muscle power can be retained by exercises, suitable games and swimming, which is particularly useful. Function can be helped by careful timing before it is lost. Plaster of paris or polythene night splints may prevent equinus deformity. A walking aid can be given just before the child ceases to walk, and this skill may be retained a little longer. A corset or spinal brace may prevent kyphoscoliosis. Lying prone for an hour a day on a foam wedge or board may delay the development of flexion contractions. Every effort must be made to practise and retain hand and finger skills. The boy will then be able to use a hand or finger-controlled electric-powered wheelchair and a typewriter.

Surgery is not usually called for. A period of immobilisation is deleterious; the child never makes up for the weakness caused by inactivity. He should be kept active as much and as long as possible. There is a danger of obesity and the diet should be watched.

The electrocardiograph may be abnormal with a high R wave. Many affected children become myopic.

A number of children with muscular dystrophy are mentally retarded. Some are at an educationally subnormal level of ability, but quite a number are severely mentally retarded. It is not unusual to see a child already in an institution for the subnormal develop muscular dystrophy. This raises the question as to whether this condition is purely a deteriorating muscle disease or whether there is not a central nervous system involvement. A proportion show an abnormal EEG.

Many boys are, however, within the normal range of intelligence, and it is extremely important that they carry on with their education at the level of their ability. For as long as possible provision should be made for them in a normal school. Later a boy may have to attend a school for the physically handicapped. Home tuition, which isolates the child, is the worst possible arrangement.

The family, and the boy himself, have to face up to the situation that there will be gradual deterioration and eventually early death. The child and the whole family can become depressed and show emotional strain. He should carry on with a lively and interesting life, with a chance to compete where he can with normal boys. The home should be a stimulating environment, with books, pets and television. The family need the regular support of a social worker, and parents have found that joining associations such as the Muscular Dystrophy Group of Great Britain has been helpful. Group discussions with similarly involved parents, under the guidance of a skilled leader, can help them to come to terms with the problem. If the boy survives school life, he will need employment which can be carried out at home, such as translating, journalism or running an agency.

Dystrophia Myotonica

This condition is inherited as an autosomal dominant with variable penetrance. One parent may show the condition in a mild form and be unaware of any abnormality. There is frequently a family history of baldness, diabetes or cataract.

There is often a history of hypotonia in the neonatal period and delay in reaching the milestones of crawling and walking. Early feeding may have been difficult due to muscle weakness, but the child usually overcomes these problems. In later childhood he has difficulty in smiling. The mouth remains half open and there is drooling. Due to the myotonic wasting of the facial muscles there is eversion of the lower eyelids and epiphora and the child is continually wiping tears away. The temporal muscles may be atrophic, making the skull appear narrow, and there is difficulty in closing the eyelids. The facial appearance of these children is quite distinct, and they can be recognised immediately (figure 16.2).

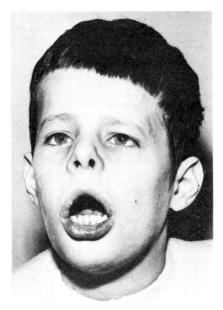

Fig. 16.2 A boy with dystrophia myotonica and a severely subnormal level of intelligence.

The form of muscular weakness is characteristic. Due to the myotonia, jerks such as the biceps jerks are prolonged, and after grasping an object, the child can only relax his grip slowly. There is noticeable atrophy of the sternomastoid muscles in the neck. Walking gradually deteriorates. The electromyogram is typical and can be used to confirm the diagnosis.

In adolescence and early adult life, myocardial involvement, lens opacities and diabetes may occur. There is gonadal atrophy in both sexes; and complete or partial infertility. People with this condition are at particular risk with anaesthesia and are liable to die of hyperthermia due to lack of temperature control. This information should be known by all persons caring for these children.

Dystrophia myotonica has been called a rare disease; but the frequent association of this condition with severe or moderate mental retardation has not often been reported. Children with the typical facies can be seen in most hospitals for the subnormal, where the condition may not have been diagnosed.

It is possible for an intelligent parent with a mild manifestation of the condition to have more severely affected mentally retarded children.

The muscular weakness is very slowly progressive, and most children live to middle age and die of diabetes, heart failure or respiratory conditions, or under anaesthetic. It is very difficult to obtain employment for them with the double handicap of mental retardation and muscle weakness.

Rheumatoid Arthritis (Still's Disease)

Some children who have had a severe illness will later attend schools for the physically handicapped. If the condition is not active, they should lead as normal a life as they are able.

The limbs should be immobilised as little as possible during the day. Night splints may be necessary to prevent fixed deformities. Physiotherapy to encourage gentle movement will help; but these children particularly benefit from hydrotherapy (figure 16.3).

More severely affected children may require crutches or a wheel-chair while continuing with a normal education.

Osteogenesis Imperfecta (Fragilitas Ossium)

This condition is due to autosomal dominant gene with variable penetrance in families. There is a tendency for the bones to fracture early due to a maldevelopment of mature collagen. Fractures may have occurred before birth and the child may be stillborn or die early, but others live on to adult life. Fractures occur easily in childhood, often by the simple action of hugging the child. The tendency to fracture gets less as the child gets older.

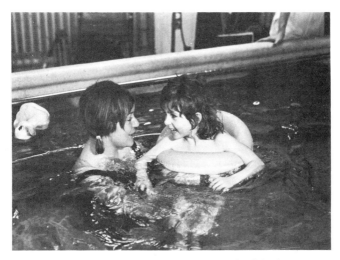

Fig. 16.3 Hydrotherapy giving a handicapped child enjoyment.

The skull in infancy is large and soft and often flattened antero-posteriorly. Apart from the deformity due to fractures the child is often dwarfed. The bones have a slender cortex and show osteoporosis. The condition is characterised by blue sclerotics which may be present in other members of the family. Deafness may develop in adult life.

Every attempt must be made to obtain a perfect union following a fracture or the child will become severely deformed. At the same time the limb should be immobilised as little as possible to prevent osteoporosis.

Intramedullary nailing of the bones has been used to prevent fractures and anabolic steroids have been given to prevent osteoporosis.

Children with this condition, although dwarfed, grossly deformed and often unable to walk, may have a normal or above average intelligence. It is important that they receive the best education of which they are capable. There is little justification for placing them in special schools for the physically handicapped, as fractures are just as likely to occur among a group of incoordinated handicapped as among normal children who will sympathetically protect the child. No particular daily therapy is needed; so the child should have an uninterrupted academic education.

MANAGEMENT

The child who becomes handicapped during school life must be sympathetically handled by the school staff, family doctor and paediatrician. The child's whole family is intimately concerned. Any arrangement for schooling must make sure that he receives the right therapy and appliances at the right time.

It is usually best for him to stay at his normal school for as long as possible, provided he can keep up with the class academically and is not unduly fatigued. If he is falling behind in school work, an opinion from a psychiatrist or psychologist may be necessary to make certain that the cause is not emotional and cannot be remedied by counselling.

If a change to a special school is considered, there should be a case conference with all concerned to decide the best type of education. If the patient himself is an older child his opinion should be considered, as he may have strong views about his own life. Resident school placing may sometimes provide a fuller social life.

If there is no mental deterioration it is imperative that the child continues with his academic education and takes all the examinations that he would have taken if unhandicapped. If this rule is not followed, he may end up an illiterate as well as a physical cripple.

If he is referred to a special school, he should stay there until the final deterioration. All appliances such as electric typewriters, the Possum machine and powered wheelchairs should be available; and there should be no question of a further placement at a hospital unit for chronically handicapped children.

HANDICAPS DUE TO
MEDICAL CONDITIONS

Medical conditions, which give rise to a need for special educational provision during childhood, such as asthma and haemophilia, are discussed in textbooks of general paediatrics. The outlook and everyday life of children with these conditions has altered dramatically due to modern treatment.

Asthma

With good home care, an allergen-reduced environment, appropriate and timely medication, and an understanding school staff, the majority of these children can attend school with their friends. The reason for placing an asthmatic child in a special school is usually a social one. Unsatisfactory home conditions and stresses within the family can aggravate the condition. Children from this type of home may suffer educationally because of frequent absences from school. Admission to a day special school such as a School for Delicate Children, where sympathetic and dynamic nursing care is provided, may be the best solution for a limited period. A school nurse can institute treatment for an attack quickly and give support to the child and the teacher. A calm attitude to the handicap may mean that the child has prolonged periods of absence from attacks.

When the attitude of the family or poor social conditions are adversely affecting the child, admission to a resident school for asthmatic children may be necessary. Children at these schools usually have fewer attacks at school than when they are home for the holidays, but deaths due to status asthmaticus do occur at school.

A resident school at Davos, Switzerland, where there is a comparatively allergen-free environment, has proved beneficial to some severely affected children and some local education authorities in Britain have taken financial responsibility for the occasional child. This may be a lifesaving measure, and hazards such as overuse of pressurised aerosols containing isoprenaline, or undue reliance on corticosteroids, which may cause dwarfing may be avoided.

Haemophilia

This is a congenital lifelong bleeding disorder. Two-thirds of the cases are genetically determined and passed on an average to 1 in 2 of the male children of an asymptomatic female carrier. In one-third of the cases there is no family history and the condition must be a new mutation. There are various forms of the disease, which are all due to an absence of an essential factor in the blood clotting mechanism. This subject is dealt with in textbooks of general paediatrics.

The disability is usually first noticed when the child is a toddler and excessive bleeding after minor accidents occurs. In later infancy haemorrhage is more likely to occur into joints and muscles due to closed injuries. A severe pain causes a sudden disinclination to use the affected limb, a limp in walking or a sleep disturbance.

Frequent haemorrhages into a joint cause thickening of the synovial membrane. This will lead to limitation of movement in the joint, contractures, and eventually osteoarthritis. The joint most commonly affected is the knee joint.

Muscle atrophy may be the end result of haemorrhage into a muscle, but disuse atrophy may also occur due to a disinclination to use the knee joint. An uneven gait, particularly due to weakening of the quadriceps muscles may lead to further damage of the knee joint and to the danger of intra-articular haemorrhages. Apart from flexion deformities of the knees, an equinus deformity in the ankle and flexion deformities in the elbows and other joints may gradually develop. Muscle atrophy and premature epiphyseal fusion may lead to stunting of growth in the limbs. A haemolytic cyst may develop in muscle tissue, which can lead to thinning of the underlying bone and fracture. Many older haemophiliacs are cripples.

Fortunately the outlook today for the younger children is much better. When bleeding is suspected, and the child can usually tell by the sensation of pain, an intravenous injection of cryoprecipitate, a product of frozen plasma, should be given within an hour. Children with haemophilia should carry a card or wear a medallion on which the details of name, address, age, blood group, type of blood deficiency, address and telephone number of the nearest treatment centre are given. This means that the child should live no further than twenty miles from a haematological unit with a casualty officer on immediate call. The prospect of a long journey to a boy in pain may be a factor in delaying attendance for treatment, and the family must be prepared to move house. Modern techniques have reduced the volume of fluid needed for an emergency intravenous injection to 30–50 ml. Experiments are taking place in the USA and in this country on home treatment. Some parents who have the use of a deep freeze for storage can be taught to give the injection at home.

The injured limb should be rested in extension with the use of a well-padded splint, such as orthoplast. With immediate treatment many children are now up and about in a few days. Movements of the affected limb can be encouraged by gentle exercises. Swimming is excellent exercise for haemophiliacs, but other formal games are contraindicated.

There is a danger of profound anaemia developing. It is important to avoid frequent injections and blood examinations in these children. An immune factor to cryoprecipitate may develop in about 3% of cases and complicate treatment. Aspirin should never be taken.

The majority can attend normal school; the school staff must be prepared to send the child to hospital if a bleed occurs. Arrangements for this eventuality must be made in advance. Home teaching during periods of absence may prevent educational delay.

Severely affected children who have frequent bleeding episodes and some deformed children may need placement at a school for delicate children or for physically handicapped children. For social reasons some children may need a resident placement in a school within the orbit of a hospital treatment centre. Several schools for haemophiliac children only have been established. In a resident school in France it was found that on average a child lost 42 school days a year due to episodes of bleeding; there must be facilities for children to make up schooltime that they are missing.

Parents need help to come to terms with the child's handicap. Refusal to accept the disability may be a reason for delay in getting immediate treatment and can be a cause of unnecessary handicap and deformity. The child has to learn to live with his handicap and to become independent. The child may expose himself to unnecessary hazards as a means of proving himself. Sympathetic handling and a lively, interesting education and social activities after school are needed to help the child accept his handicap.

REFERENCES

BODER E & SEDGWICK R P (1958) Ataxia telangiectasia. *Pediatrics*, **21**, 526

CALDERON R (1966) Myotonic dystrophy. A neglected cause of mental retardation. *J. Pediat.* **68**, 423

CRAFT A W, SHAW D A & CARTLIDGE N E F (1972) Head injuries in children. *Brit. med. J.* **4**, 200

FORD F R (1960) *Diseases of the Nervous System in Infancy, Childhood and Adolescence.* Blackwell, Oxford

GAMSTORP I (1969) *Paediatric Neurology.* Appleton-Century Crofts, New York

KIERMANDER B (1965) *Physical Medicine in Paediatrics.* Butterworth, London

MEALEY J (1968) *Paediatric Head Injuries.* C C Thomas, Illinois

MILLICHAP J G & DODGE P R (1960) Diagnosis and treatment of myasthenia gravis in infancy, childhood and adolescence. *Neurology (Minneap.)* **10**, 1007

MUSCULAR DYSTROPHY GROUPS OF GREAT BRITAIN. London

PICKARD K A, MACDONALD D, GREGG S, BELLAMY A & KERR C B (1972) *Haemophilia. Proc. 12th World Congress of Rehabilitation International, Sydney, Australia*

SPENCER G U (1972) *Mobile units in rural areas. Proc. 12th World Congress of Rehabilitation International, Sydney, Australia,* p. 837

WALTON J N & GARDNER-MEDWIN D (1968) Second thoughts on the classification of muscular dystrophy. *4th Symposium on Current Research in Muscular Dystrophy, London*

Chapter 17
General Considerations

The preceding chapters have emphasised the need for a team approach in the assessment and management of a handicapped child. To work in a team, each member must fully appreciate the role of every other member and his own place in the team.

In the early years the parents, the paediatricians, the family doctor, the health visitors and the therapists may be the most important people in the child's care. Very early in his life the local social services and the education authorities have a part to play, and their role increases as he gets older. In the clinical care and the treatment it is important for him that there should be one doctor who takes the responsibility for organising medical care for him. If the child is under many doctors there is the danger that no one will take the ultimate responsibility and the parents will not know to which doctor to turn to discuss the total picture. One doctor should feel that the clinical condition, functional ability and emotional status of a handicapped child, when school age is reached, have been his responsibility. It is becoming generally recognised that this doctor should be a paediatrician; and he should lead the team in all matters associated with the clinical care of the child.

INFANCY

Early Paediatric Consultation

The parents of a handicapped child often make their first contact with a paediatrician in the neonatal period, either because there is a congenital abnormality, or because the child is severely ill after birth and there is a danger of cerebral damage. If an abnormality is noticed at birth, the parents should be told immediately. It is important that both parents should hear about the deformity from a doctor and it is not a task that should be left to a midwife or a nurse or discovered by the mother on first seeing her child. The paediatrician who will have the future supervision of the child or the family doctor should have a preliminary talk with the parents. Both parents should be told together, and neither should be given the job of telling the other.

If permission is needed for immediate operation, the doctor must judge how much he can tell the parents; but with the present television coverage of problems of handicapped children, many parents will have some background knowledge. The final decision to recommend immediate surgery or palliative measures only must be a medical one. Years later, when a child is severely handicapped, the parents should not be left with feelings of guilt that they made the decision that this child should live.

Follow-up Clinic

After the first discussions the paediatrician should make an appointment to see the parents a week or two later. By then they will have many questions to ask and they should be encouraged to talk and verbalise their worries. They will want to know about the child's likely intelligence and future schooling, and whether he will earn his living. Many of these questions are difficult to answer, but the truth or lack of knowledge must always be told. The first discussion that the parents have with a doctor is often indelibly printed on their minds, and in later years will continue to assume tremendous importance. A path must be steered between undue optimism and undue pessimism.

Sometimes, as in the case of children with Down's syndrome (mongolism), a fairly definite picture can be given. It is possible to let the parents see older mongols in a school or in a workshop. A mother with a 6 week old mongol was surprised and reassured when shown an adult mongol working in a hospital laundry.

The parents usually want to know about the possibility of having further affected children. Simple genetic advice can be given at this stage and arrangements can be made for a later referral to a Genetic Clinic.

The mother of a congenitally deformed child needs regular support in these early months as she may become depressed and find it difficult to show pride and affection for her child. She may isolate herself from her friends and find it difficult to face up to their interest and to the stares of strangers, and although giving good physical care to the baby she may give little stimulation. A social worker or health visitor with an insight into the mother's problems may be the ideal person to visit the home and help her at this stage. The father may be feeling intense disappointment as he may look upon the birth of the handicapped child, particularly a son, as a slur on his masculinity and he also needs support. The child with his family must be seen regularly by the paediatrician.

Later Diagnosis of Abnormality

In many instances the handicap is only revealed when the child is late in attaining early baby skills. The child's name may be on the local 'at risk' register, but often the parents are the first to worry about his delayed development. Every concern by parents should be taken seriously as they are usually right. They should not be allowed to worry without an avenue of obtaining advice.

The health visitor, the family doctor or the infant welfare clinic doctor may be the recipient of the parents' worries, and if there is any concern the child should see a paediatrician.

Assessment Centre

It has been emphasised that the majority of handicapped children today are multiply handicapped. It is also stressed that a handicap should be investigated early, both to give the family support and to start treatment. To carry out this work satisfactorily, purpose-built centres should be set up on a district and regional basis. The Sheldon Report (1967) emphasised the need for these centres and suggested that they should be hospital based. Others have suggested that the centres should be community based and associated with local health and education services. Possibly a hospital based service is needed for the very young child before he reaches nursery school age.

At the Assessment Centre the full history, investigation and assessments are made. Whilst the clinic may be under one specially appointed paediatrician with all paramedical services provided, it would also be of value if paediatricians with a particular interest in one condition held clinics and took the responsibility for children with these handicaps, e.g. mental retardation, epilepsy or spina bifida.

Ongoing Assessment

As has been stressed a full assessment cannot be made at one visit and there is a need for ongoing assessment. The Centre staff should have facilities by which a child with or without a parent can attend for observation in a play-orientated environment. The information obtained from the therapists by this prolonged observation can form a basis for decisions on future school placement, and the services of a nursery school teacher at the Centre would be valuable.

Treatment

In official discussions on Assessment Centres insufficient emphasis has been laid on arrangements for early treatment. Parents can become extremely angry if assessment alone is offered and no facilities for treatment are arranged. Active measures must be made to ensure that the child gets treatment either at the Centre or near his home. This may involve communication between therapists at outlying clinics or arrangements for domiciliary treatment. Sometimes the mother must be the therapist and be instructed in her role. She should return to the Centre at frequent intervals to ensure that she understands what to do. This latter arrangement has worked extremely well with some parents and not so well with others.

Information Service

The Assessment Centre should be the source of information about treatment, appliances, aids to daily living and literature on all handicaps. Lectures and courses for all grades of staff should be held and the paediatrician in charge should take a keen interest in the training of all personnel dealing with handicapped children. Accurate records should be kept at the Centre which can be used for research, for establishing local incidence of a particular handicap, and for giving advanced warning of early educational needs.

Cooperation with Education Authorities

Staff at the Assessment Centres for handicapped children should have direct contact with the authorities arranging for education. Ideally educationists of whatever profession should visit the Centre and observe the children while they are having group play or therapy, and decisions on future education should be made after case conferences with the Assessment Centre staff.

Follow-up Clinics

Parents with a handicapped baby do not usually wish to attend an infant welfare clinic where the child's abnormality and delayed milestones become increasingly obvious. It is preferable if children with a handicap can attend a clinic tailormade for their require-ments. At these clinics parents should obtain advice about feeding, dressing and toileting. Therapists of all three categories should be available to advise, and treatment for conditions such as epilepsy should be given. Parents can discuss problems such as how to tell the other children about the handicapped child and how to deal with the attitudes of in-laws, of neighbours and of neighbours' children. They may want advice on play and toys. A clinic of this type can be held at the Assessment Centre; but the numbers of handicapped children are so great that clinics strategically placed in the community with the services of a social worker and therapists are necessary.

The value of these clinics has been illustrated by a clinic intended for children under 5 years, where parents were still bringing 18 year old handicapped children.

Social Worker

In team work with parents a social worker has a particular role, and a report on the home is an essential piece of information. The doctor needs to know the facilities at home for caring for the child. It is important to know the attitudes of all members of the family and the type of support the mother is getting from them. The social worker can iron out all kinds of problems, explain to the parents information given by the paediatrician that they do not understand and relay back information about misconceptions. The social worker can also help with the physical needs of the family, either a need for financial help, alteration in the structure of the home or the supply of appliances.

Home Visits by Therapists

Much benefit may accrue from home visits by the therapists. The physiotherapist can see what type of chair, walking aid or appliances are possible in a particular home. An occupational therapist can go into the problem of toileting, feeding, bathing and play, and see what apparatus and alterations to the home are necessary. Speech therapists can give advice on feeding the child in the home situation, and can encourage the mother to stimulate early language.

Toys for the Handicapped

There has been a considerable amount of research on suitable toys for handicapped children, and literature is available (Nottingham University 1972). In some areas there are toy libraries for the handicapped, and well-planned toys can be borrowed for short periods. Toys are needed for very young handicapped babies to encourage use of both hands and to encourage hand-eye coordination. For older children there must be large mobility toys, constructional toys with a recognisable end product, and toys which encourage creative activity. Other toys must develop powers of discrimination and skills in speech, language, number and music.

The Mother

Emotional support must be given to the mother and the family from the first realisation that the child is handicapped, and throughout the child's early development, until they have come to terms with the situation. The mother's early feelings of guilt, shame, anxiety and rejection must be understood.

A physical handicap in a baby will delay the development of a happy social interchange between the mother and the baby. A blind baby will not smile at his mother or later reach for toys that she offers. A deaf child may take no notice when she enters a room and will not respond to verbal endearments. A child with a severe motor handicap may be unresponsive due to poor head control and an inability to control his arm and hand movements. A mentally retarded child will have an overall delay in understanding his environment, and show a general lack of response.

Children who are deprived of a means to explore compensate by excessive involvement with their own bodies, and mannerisms such as the body-rocking and eye-poking of the blind child may develop. The abnormal significance of bodily functions to the child may lead to a refusal to alter routine. The mother of a handicapped child often finds it difficult to change the child on to new foods, and more than usually difficult to institute toilet training and regular sleeping patterns. A change of routine will more easily arouse temper tantrums than in a normal child, and the child may realise that he can dominate his family circle by his screaming attacks.

The handicapped child may not give clues to his mother that he is ready for the next stage of development; and a caring mother may be unwittingly holding him back and keeping him too long at a dependent baby stage.

If the child is both physically and mentally retarded the mother's task is even more difficult. A mentally retarded child may be late in learning to chew and drink from a cup as part of the general backwardness. If his overall understanding is behind that of a normal child, the mother will have problems in organising play, instituting discipline and arranging social contacts with other children.

Mothers react in different ways to these problems. Possibly all of them at some time have subconscious feelings of guilt and go through periods of rejecting the child. Some mothers become overtly depressed; and this further delays the child's development.

How these attitudes affect the mother and the family must be understood by the health visitor, social worker and therapists. It is important that at all times the mother is treated as an intelligent person, and that she is not made to feel more inadequate than she feels already. To point out mistakes that the mother is making in handling her child may only make her feel more insecure. The help given to the mother, although basically psychotherapeutic, does not usually need the services of a psychiatrist, and may be resented. As one mother said to me: 'I may have a batty child, but that does not mean I am batty myself'.

Efficient help for the child's physical needs and therapy in a happy play environment may go a long way towards helping the mother to achieve a balanced attitude to her problems. Nothing is so therapeutic as progress in the child. Knowing where to obtain immediate help with her many problems can ease the family problem; and a secure knowledge of the way ahead for treatment and education can help the family to face up to the situation.

The Family

A family with a handicapped child is a handicapped family. Many normal activities such as outings and holidays are curtailed. The siblings may be deprived of their mother's attention, and often parents may be overdemanding of their normal children, as if they are trying to prove that they are capable of having a 'perfect' child. The sibling of a handicapped child may be more emotionally disturbed than the child himself.

There is a serious danger of a break up of the marriage unless it is founded on firm mutual respect between the parents. The mother must be helped to understand the disappointment of her husband, who also needs support. It is not uncommon to find that after a very handicapped child has died, or been placed in an institution, the marriage breaks up. The father has done his duty admirably, but because of the strain, affection and love have gone out of the marriage and the father feels he no longer has a duty to his wife.

PRESCHOOL YEARS (2–5)

It is hoped that children with a handicap can join a play group or a nursery school at the age of 3 years. This is particularly important for children with a severe hearing loss, who need early training in spoken language; but it is also important for the blind, the physically handicapped and the mentally handicapped. The handicapped child of 3 years needs all the play experience of a normal child. He should have a chance to play with sand and water, to paint and to play in gangs. This is the age when the mother needs some day relief from the care of the child, particularly if he is not yet walking. By this age many mothers have or are expecting another child.

A handicapped child may attend a nursery school with unhandicapped children, but this situation wants careful supervision. An adult must see that the child is able physically to benefit from the play equipment, has the right type of chair and equipment for mobility, and is allowed to explore the play environment fully. If this way of catering for the young handicapped child is the method of choice in any area a peripatetic qualified person, possibly a therapist, should go round the play groups to supervise the handicapped children.

There are many cases when special nursery units for severely handicapped units are preferable. The child can play in an environment tailormade for his needs, and at the same time receive supervision and regular therapy from a physiotherapist, speech therapist and occupational therapist.

Role of Psychologist

At the age of 5 years in Britain, and at 6–7 years in some other countries, formal education begins. The member of the team who should have a final say in the type of education that a particular child needs is the psychologist. In some countries such as Britain a doctor has made these decisions, and in other countries such as the USA and the Scandinavian countries it is the psychologist. This latter arrangement puts the emphasis on the educational needs of the child and not on the needs of his physical handicap, and may be the more appropriate approach.

A psychologist should see the child regularly in his preschool years; and should have watched the progress he has made in language, performance skills and problem solving. The psychologist's task nowadays is not considered as one of giving the clinician a numerical intelligence quotient with which to label the child. He should have used his battery of tests and his own observations to understand the child's problems and abilities. These tests should be a means to help him and not merely to assess him. A very young handicapped child cannot be compared on any scale with a normal child. This is obvious under 2 years of age with the Griffiths and Sheridan scales. In later childhood the child's organic difficulties, lack of everyday experiences and organically determined learning problems interfere with the performance of a large number of the recognised intelligence tests. The more handicapped the child, the less easily can he be compared with a normal child of the same age. The child's innate intelligence may have little relationship to the degree of physical handicap. A severely handicapped child may have an intelligence above average, and an apparently mildly handicapped child may have a low intelligence.

The psychologist must assess the child not on what he can do but on how well he can learn if he is put in a learning situation. By assessing how a child can solve a problem the psychologist can forecast his future ability to learn educational skills. This is the basis of the Piaget method of assessment. Advice can then be given as to the type of school for which the child is ready, and the correct approach needed to teach him.

SCHOOL YEARS

It is important that the handicapped child should receive the best education of which he is capable; and his physical handicap should not mean that he has less opportunity. If the handicap is not caused by brain pathology, he should receive a normal education, with no unnecessary rest periods and other hindrances to normal schooling.

Ferguson & Kerr (1960) have said, 'Lack of education may dominate a youth's future, even when the original cause of disability has largely disappeared'. Every effort should be made to educate the child with his normal friends. This method has been tried with the blind, partially sighted, hard of hearing and physically handicapped. In Sweden, physically handicapped children are helped in normal classes by the provision of a personal assistant. She helps the child with transport round the school and with toileting but works the minimum number of hours to prevent him from becoming over dependent. This method is actually cheaper than attendance with the cost of individual transport at a special school. In parts of the USA peripatetic 'resource' teachers visit the schools where there is a handicapped child in a class to help him with any extra tuition or assistance that is needed, and special 'resource' rooms are set aside for this purpose. Developing countries such as Iran and some African countries are using this method of education, particularly for the blind. It has been said that blind children make more progress and hard of hearing children develop more language by this method. The education of a handicapped child in a normal class was the theme of the Fifth International Seminar on Special Education held in 1972 in Melbourne, Australia.

Children with a more severe physical handicap, particularly if they need aids such as an electric typewriter, may not fit into a normal class. It is suggested that special classes for these children should be on the same campus as a normal school, so that the children can join with their peers whenever possible. In Sweden, a school for 600 children has 6 classes for 10 handicapped of each age level (6–16 years). Thus 10% of the school is a handicapped population but the total environment is that of school for unhandicapped children.

Where there are specific learning problems, special programmes of education are needed and non-physically handicapped children with a learning problem require a special class. The numbers of these children are so great that many day schools could provide the necessary facilities in 'slow learning', 'progress' or 'remedial' classes. A child with a physical handicap and a learning problem will need periods of individual tuition, as may a hyperactive, distractible child.

There will be children who because of home circumstances and the distance of a special school from home will need resident school placement. It is hoped that these schools will be on a Monday to Friday basis, with transport home at weekends.

Possibly a fair percentage of handicapped children would benefit from residential schooling at 11–13 years of age when they can be weaned away from over dependence on parents. It is at this age that a non-ambulant child may become too heavy for a mother to handle.

Schools for Delicate Children

The Department of Education and Science in Britain defines a group of handicapped children as 'delicate pupils: that is to say pupils not falling under any other category, who by reason of impaired physical condition need a change of environment or cannot without risk to their health or educational development be educated under the normal regime of ordinary schools'.

Children with a wide variety of conditions could fit into this category; and the list of conditions includes:

a Asthma, particularly where the condition is aggravated by unfavourable home circumstances.

b Cystic fibrosis, where regular physiotherapy for postural lung drainage is required and physically the child cannot cope with the strain of normal school.

c Bronchiectasis, after recent surgery.

d A mild physical handicap but marked learning and behaviour problems following a cerebral injury.

e Intractable eczema.

f Inoperable congenital heart defects.

g Severe haemophilia associated with frequent bleeding episodes.

h An ileostomy which the child cannot manage himself.

j Maladjustment manifesting itself by school refusal, elective mutism, withdrawn and passive behaviour.

(Children with aggressive and acting-out behaviour are more correctly placed in a school for maladjusted children.)

This wide variety of handicapped and deprived children may be found today in a special school, which in the past was designated as 'Open-Air School' and catered for children with tuberculosis, the after effects of rheumatic fever and malnutrition.

School medical officers, educational psychologists and administrators have a difficult task arranging suitable education for the above group of children. Placement of an intelligent child with a chronic illness but no specific learning handicap in a school with non-mobile children requiring special educational techniques and appliances may not be appropriate. Some authorities have found that all the above categories can mix in one school. Each child must be treated as an individual and the staff-pupil ratio must be high. A trained nurse is an essential member of the staff.

The establishment of a small school of this type may solve many educational problems, and give short-term or longterm placement to a few children who are difficult to place and can attend on a daily basis. A paediatrician and a child psychiatrist should be actively involved in such a school and support the teaching staff and the nurse dealing with children who are constantly requiring medical care. If the school is situated near a hospital for children, the staff will feel that they can readily get help if they admit a particularly ill child.

Return to Normal School

With help in a special school many children will improve and can later be transferred back to a normal school, so the decision to send a young child to a special school need not mean special schooling for life. Possibly a handicapped child may benefit from nursery and infant school life in a special school, and later education in a normal school where he learns to live with the unhandicapped. The seriousness of the physical handicap may change with growing up.

Experience of the Outside World

During these formative years the child should have every opportunity to get around and see the world outside his immediate environment. A method used in Sweden can be recommended. Handicapped children with a parent (and handicapped adults) are allowed to travel fifteen miles by taxi free at any time. The cost of the taxi is obtained from State monies and in this way travel to school and all hospital appointments are easily arranged and the child can take part in a normal social life. The actual cost may not be greater than our present inefficient transport and ambulance service (because of too much demand) and the child can have independence in his own right.

Sporting and Recreational Facilities

If a handicapped child cannot join in normal games such as football, an alternative should be found. Every area should have an adventure playground for the handicapped. Swimming and horse riding are excellent recreations for many handicapped children, archery has been found suitable for wheelchair-bound children and wheelchair hockey and dances can be arranged. Emphasis on music and appreciation of art in school will give the child enjoyment throughout life and make him eligible for admission to many adult activities when he leaves school, and handicapped children should be able to attend youth clubs.

Medical Care

During his school life there must be regular supervision and the therapists have an important part to play. The school doctor must be a paediatrician with a profound knowledge of all types of handicapping conditions, both relatively common handicaps and rare syndromes, so that all children are given the appropriate treatment and advice. He should be able to appreciate when the child needs the help of the child psychiatrist. Every appliance that will help independence should be available and the therapists must work with the teachers, who should be as interested in the child's attainment of daily living skills as in his general education. Children have been known to have advanced educational knowledge and yet are not independent on the toilet, when this skill should be readily attained. This situation will arise unless a broad view of what education for life really means. If the teacher has not the time or facilities to train the child to feed, wash, dress and toilet himself, she must allow the access to her class of a therapist, particularly an occupational therapist, for the training of these skills, and this dual approach to education has often worked very well.

Emotional Problems

Teachers, therapists and house parents working with handicapped children during their school years have been surprised by the comparative absence of emotional disturbances. This is particularly true if the child has led a happy early childhood, and has no unpleasant memories of treatment. These children have received so much individual attention that they may not feel the need to be attention seeking, or to dominate their family circle by tantrums of temper. Some of these children have been described as 'too good'. Certainly a large number of handicapped children enjoy their school life and activities and accept their disabilities. Problems may arise when they cannot attend evening clubs and other teenage activities, and every effort must be made to provide this.

The self-image of the child must be altered if he has had long periods of hospitalisation and painful operative procedures. The child may then look upon himself as an ill child, be passive in his attitudes and expect the world to take over responsibility for his life. Hospitalisation should be reduced to a minimum, and reasons for surgical procedures discussed with the child.

Gradually the handicapped schoolchild will realise how his handicap will affect his future life, chances of employment and marriage. Direct discussions on his handicap should be introduced into conversations at school and at home; and false hopes that the child is fostering should be corrected quietly and immediately. Children may want to ask about the likelihood of independent walking, or being able to drive a car. Staff must not be frightened of tackling a conversation of this type. The school staff may arrange talks for the children on job opportunities. Suitable children may be taken on a visit to a work centre for handicapped children, or shown a bungalow specially adapted for handicapped people.

Handicapped children of this age rarely need the direct help of a psychiatrist or attendance at a child guidance clinic. There should be a psychiatrist available to support the school and therapeutic staff, and possibly to attend case conferences to give advice on the best way to tackle each situation as it arises.

The incidence of behaviour problems due to a physical handicap become progressively more evident as the level of intelligence gets lower, and there are more problems in children with an educationally subnormal level of intelligence. The abnormalities in behaviour of the severely subnormal child may require the understanding of an interested psychiatrist, and special psychotherapeutic measures such as behaviour modification or drug therapy.

Employment

At the end of school life, handicapped adolescents must be fitted for life in the community. Intense individual training in special schools may not have prepared them to live independently, and some leave school immature and self-centred. For many children there is a need for further education after the age of 16 years to encourage self-reliance. Various voluntary organisations in England, such as the Royal National Institute for the Blind and the Spastics Society, run courses for school leavers where independence on transport, self-care and work habits are taught.

Some adolescents leave school to attend further training courses at special day or resident units, and this is often the best method of ensuring that they will get a worthwhile job. Some may leave school and be able to obtain a job without this help and some will go on to further education and university. Others may only be able to work in a sheltered workshop or work centre.

The doctor who has looked after the child during his school life should be present at a school leavers' conference where decisions as to further placement are made. Information such as treatment for fits and the need for regular urine testing in spina bifida must be passed on to doctors at resident units or to Industrial Medical Officers.

There is often a serious break in medical services at this age; and it is at this point in his life that the handicapped youth particularly needs support and may need more sophisticated aids. Appliances such as power-driven wheelchairs or the Possum should be arranged at the appropriate age.

Sexual Advice

Handicapped people are normal people in every way apart from their handicap. In adolescence they will go through the same emotional turmoils and indecisions and doubts about sexual matters. It is quite illogical to deny this or to hope that because the youth is handicapped the problems will not arise, and education in sex matters must be given in special schools or classes. The youth should be encouraged to verbalise his worries about marriage opportunities and sensible discussion, often in groups, must take place. The handicapped must know how they are placed with regard to any genetic hazard. Eventually the decision to marry or to have sexual experience must be taken by the handicapped adolescent himself. It is hoped that with the education and help he has been given, a mature and happy decision on a matter which intimately affects his own future will be made.

Architecture

In the Chronically Sick and Disabled Persons Act (1970) in Britain, a duty was laid on local authorities to 'ensure that premises open to the public have access and facilities for the handicapped'. There is also a need to make homes where handicapped people live suitable for them. The American Standards Association Inc (1961) have published standards for buildings, ramps, doorways, stairs, toilets, door handles etc. which are convenient for disabled people and wheelchair users. The specifications are very simple and inexpensive and in the planning of schools, colleges, restaurants and concert halls a little extra thought is needed and all these facilities will be available to the handicapped. Voluntary organisations such as Rehabilitation International are pressing for these provisions.

ROLE OF VOLUNTARY SERVICES OR GOVERNMENT HELP

In many parts of the world the care and education of the handicapped are financed entirely by voluntary sources. To obtain the money appeal has to be made to the emotions of the general public and this attitude to the handicapped is not necessarily in his best interests. In other countries the government makes itself entirely or partly responsible for the services needed.

Many governments have fragmented legislation on the care of handicapped people. In Britain legislation is used to give powers and permission to local authorities to spend money on services for the handicapped in various ways and at different ages. This means that money to help the handicapped does not all come out of the same administrative purse. The care of the child for the first two to three years is divided between the hospital services, social services and local health authority. Sometime in the first five years of life the local education authorities take over from the local health authorities. If the child goes into permanent resident care he will be the financial responsibility of the social services or the hospital services; and the same division occurs after school age. The authority who pays for services for the young child has no administrative responsibility for him when he is an adult and the official staff may have little insight into how money used on services for the child in early life can so improve his condition that money is saved later on. It might be an advantage if at all ages the care of the handicapped, whether by local health and education, hospital or social services, was under one administrative authority.

*

The author is intensely grateful that she has had the opportunity to work with handicapped adults and watch many handicapped children grow up to adulthood. It is only with this experience that one can realise how worthwhile is the early management and treatment suggested in this book.

REFERENCES

BAILEY C H (1968) *The Characteristics and Needs of Delicate Children. What is Special Education?* p. 97. Association of Special Education, Middlesex

BETOVIM A (1972) Handicapped pre-school children and their families. *Brit. med. J.* **3**, 634

BRITISH COUNCIL FOR REHABILITATION OF THE DISABLED (1963) *The Handicapped School Leaver.* Tavistock House, London

CARNEGIE UNITED KINGDOM TRUST (1964) *Handicapped Children and Their Families.* Constable, Edinburgh

FERGUSON T & KERR A W (1960) *Handicapped Youth.* Oxford University Press, London

FROSTIG M (1968) *Education for Children with Learning Disabilities.* Grune & Stratton, New York

GUNSBURG H G (1963) *Progress Assessment Charts.* NAMH, London

HEAD J & NEWSOM E (1971) *Toys and Handicap.* National Fund for Research into Crippling Diseases, London

ICTA INFORMATION CENTRE. Fack, Bromma 3, Sweden

INFORMATION SERVICE FOR THE DISABLED. London SW1

JAMES F E (1970) *Educational Medicine.* Heinemann, London

MEMORANDUM ON COMPREHENSIVE ASSESSMENT CENTRES (1968) HMSO, London

MITTLER P ed. (1970) *The Psychological Assessment of Mental and Physical Handicaps.* Methuen, London

MITTLER P (1971) *Purposes and Principles of Assessment.* Ciba Foundation Study Group, No. 5 London

NATIONAL SOCIETY FOR CRIPPLED CHILDREN AND ADULTS *Self Help Clothing for Handicapped Children.* 2023 West Ogden Avenue, Chicago 12, Illinois

NEWSON J & NEWSON E (1967) *Handicapped Children and their Families.* University of Nottingham, Nottingham

DEPARTMENT OF EDUCATION & SCIENCE (1971) *Physical Education for the Physically Handicapped.* HMSO, London

RUTTER M, TIZARD J & WHITMORE K (1970) *Education, Health and Behaviour.* Longman, London

SEEBOHM REPORT (1968) *Local Authority and Allied Personal Social Services.* HMSO, London

SHELDON REPORT (1967) HMSO, London

SMITH N J (1972) *A Brief Guide to Social Legislation.* Methuen, London

SMITH N J (1972) *Sports and Open Air Facilities.* Methuen, London

STONE J & TAYLOR F (1972) *Handbook for Parents with a Handicapped Child.* Home & School Council Pub., London

WILLIAMS C E (1969) *Psychiatric Implications of Severe Visual Defect for the Child and for the Parents,* p. 110. *Clinics in Developmental Medicine,* No. 32 Spastics Society & William Heinemann, London

YOUNGHUSBAND E *et al* eds. (1970) *Living with a Handicap.* National Children's Bureau, London

Nottingham University Toy Library NUTL/1
Addresses for Advice NUTL/5
Reading for Parents NUTL/5
Noah's Ark Toy Libraries for Children with Handicap (1971) London
Making Facilities Accessible to the Physically Handicapped (1967) State University
    Construction Fund. Albany, New York
What is Special Education? (1968)
Handicapped Children in Pre-School Groups (1971) *Brit. med. J*, 4561

Addresses of Voluntary Societies in Britain

Associations for Handicapped Children and their Parents

Association for all Speech-Impaired Children (AFASIC), 9 Desenfans Road, London SE21 (01-693 8670)

Association for Spina Bifida and Hydrocephalus, 112 City Road, London EC1 (01-253 2735)

British Epilepsy Association, 3–6 Alfred Place, London WC1E 7EE (01-580 2704)

Lady Hoare Trust for Thalidomide and other Physically Disabled Children, 78 Hamilton Terrace, London NW8 (01-289 0231)

Muscular Dystrophy Group of Great Britain, 26 Borough High Street, London SE1 (01-407 5116)

National Association for Deaf/Blind and Rubella Children, 61 Senneleys Park Road, Birmingham 31 (021-475 1392)

National Deaf Children's Society, 31 Gloucester Place, London W1 (01-486 3251)

National Society for Autistic Children, 1a Golders Green Road, London NW11 (01-458 4375)

National Society for Brain-Damaged Children, 35 Larchmere Drive, Hall Green, Birmingham 31 (021-777 4284)

National Society for Mentally Handicapped Children, 86 Newman Street, London W1P 4AR (01-636 2861)

Royal National Institute for the Blind, 224 Great Portland Street, London W1 (01-387 5251)

Spastics Society, 12 Park Crescent, London W2 (01-636 5020)

Information Sources

Association for Special Education, Beaconwood, Bordon Hill, Stratford-upon-Avon, Warwickshire

Disabled Living Foundation, 346 Kensington High Street, London W14 8NS (01-602 2491)

Department of Health and Social Security (Information Division), Alexander Fleming House, Elephant and Castle, London SE1 (01-407 5522)

National Children's Bureau, 1 Fitzroy Square, London W1P 5AH (01-387 4263)

Royal National Institute for the Deaf Library, 105 Gower Street, London WC1 (01-387 8033)

Spastics Society Information Service, 16 Fitzroy Square, London W1P 5HQ (01-387 9571)

General

Association of Occupational Therapists, 251 Brompton Road, London SW3 (01-589 7458)

Breakthrough Trust (for deaf and hearing), 19 Beaconfield Road, New Malden, Surrey

Chartered Society of Physiotherapy, 14 Bedford Row, London WC1 (01-242 1941)

College of Speech Therapists, 47 St Johns Wood High Street, London NW8 (01-586 1958)

Down's Babies Centre (for mongol babies), 40 Lodge Hill Road, Birmingham B29 6NG (021-472 0881)

Invalid Children's Aid Association (all handicaps and with a special interest in language disorders), 126 Buckingham Palace Road, London SW1 (01-730 9891)

National Association for the Welfare of Children in Hospital, 74 Denison House, Vauxhall Bridge Road, London SW1 (01-834 1124)

National Fund for Research into Crippling Diseases, Vincent House, Vincent Square, London SW1 (01-834 7001)

Nursery School Association, 89 Stamford Street, London SE1 (01-928 7454)

Pre-school Playgroups Association, 87a Borough High Street, London SE1 (01-407 7815)

Riding for the Disabled Association, c/o British Horse Society, National Equestrian Centre, Stoneleigh, Kenilworth, Warwickshire

Save the Children Fund, 29 Queen Anne's Gate, London SW1 (01-930 2461)

Toy Library Association, 21 Gentleman's Row, Enfield, Middlesex (01-363 1394)

Word Blind Centre for Dyslexic Children, Coram Fields, 93 Guilford Street, London WC1 (01-837 8914)

Index